Step by Step®
Management of Male Infertility

Step by Step® Management of Male Infertility

Manish R Pandya MD, FICOG
Associate Professor
CU Shah Medical College
Surendranagar, Gujarat
India

Sudhir R Shah MD DGO, FICOG
Head of Obstetrics and Gynecology Department
Dasha Shrimali Hospital
Kotharia Naka, Rajkot, Gujarat (India)

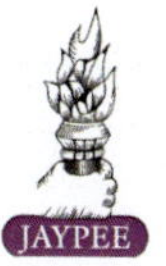

JAYPEE BROTHERS MEDICAL PUBLISHERS
The Health Sciences Publisher
New Delhi | London

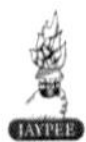

Jaypee Brothers Medical Publishers (P) Ltd

Headquarters
EMCA House
23/23-B, Ansari Road, Daryaganj
New Delhi 110 002, India
Landline: +91-11-23272143, +91-11-23272703
+91-11-23282021, +91-11-23245672
E-mail: jaypee@jaypeebrothers.com

Corporate Office
4838/24, Ansari Road, Daryaganj
New Delhi 110 002, India
Phone: +91-11-43574357
Fax: +91-11-43574314
E-mail: jaypee@jaypeebrothers.com

Overseas Office
J.P. Medical Ltd
83 Victoria Street, London
SW1H 0HW (UK)
Phone: +44 20 3170 8910
E-mail: info@jpmedpub.com

EU GPSR Authorised Representative
Logos Europe, 9 rue Nicolas Poussin
17000, La Rochelle, France
Phone: +33 (0) 6 67 93 73 78
E-mail: contact@logoseurope.eu

Website: www.jaypeebrothers.com
Website: www.jaypeedigital.com

Inquiries for bulk sales may be solicited at: jaypee@jaypeebrothers.com

Step by Step® Management of Male Infertility

First Edition: 2008
Reprint: **2026**
ISBN 978-81-8448-314-7
Printed at: Samrat Offset Pvt. Ltd.

To

Our Patients
Who kept full faith in us and
Encouraged us indirectly
to write
This small booklet.

Our family members
Without whose constant inspiration
and
Cooperation
This attempt would not have been completed.

FOREWORD

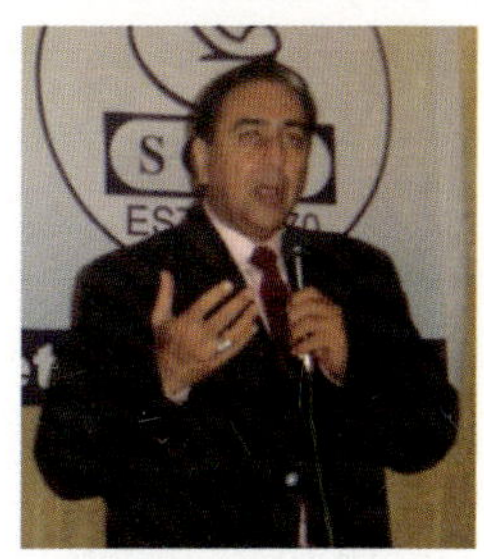

Dr Jayant Mehta

It is indeed a pleasure and an honour for me to write a Foreword for this extremely informative and much needed reference guide on Male infertility. As a result of the rapid development of *in vitro* fertilization (IVF) for treating both male and female infertility, male infertility has become just as important for a consultant gynecologist assessing an infertile couple as it has for a specialist andrologist. Consequently, the detailed and intricate tests that consultant andrologist developed to identify the cause of male infertility and proposed treatments have drifted into the clinical realm of consultant gynecologists who need to assess couples rather than simply infertile women.

Infertility is believed to affect some 60–80 million couples worldwide. This guide is intended to be a practical, accessible guide to male infertility and its treatments. Dr Sudhir R Shah and Dr Manish Pandya have ensured that the sequence of the chapters is logical. The first chapter provide an overview of anatomy and reproductive physiology of male, in particular the importance of sperm as related to fertilization. Next come chapters on the causes of male infertility and the clinical evaluation of the infertile couple, medical surgical management. These are followed by chapters describing techniques of assisted reproduction including intrauterine insemination (IUI), with both husband and donor sperm, intra-cytoplasm sperm injection (ICSI), alluding to surgical sperm retrieval. Newer drugs, currently being used are also discussed. There is a final chapter on the practical aspects of semen examination which, I believe to be the most important chapter of the text as correct and accurate semen analysis will make a difference between patients being subjected to an ICSI cycle as opposed to a simple IUI cycle.

The guide has an aesthetic appeal from its content and layout to its illustrations and diagrams. The judicious use of photographs for diagnostic procedures and surgery enhances the understanding of these sections. There are many illustrations—almost every page has a photograph or diagram. Perhaps the greatest attribute is the completeness in addressing topics relating to male infertility. Most chapters deliver a succinct, focused approach.

The chapters on treatments all have a brief conclusion in which Dr Sudhir and Dr Manish assess the contribution of the treatment. Those with basic knowledge about reproductive physiology will probably skim the first few chapters, but from Chapter 4 (on evaluation of the infertile couple) onwards both authors' expertise comes to the fore. They stress the importance of carrying out investigations that do not waste what may be precious time to the couple, and demonstrate how delays are unnecessary since all of the basic infertility investigations can take place within 1 month.

I congratulate both Dr Sudhir and Dr Manish for being very meticulous on sections describing treatments include step by step instructions for the procedures, including a sometimes surprising level of details. Their vision as stated in their Preface is that there are "institutional as well as regional differences in the manner of evaluating and treating infertile couples" and hope that these will diminish when evidence-based protocols become more widely used.

I am sure that medical students, residents, fellows, and clinicians will find this guide very helpful. Perhaps the greatest benefit is for fellows and clinicians, since the level of detail probably exceeds that needed for medical students and residents. However, the interested student or resident should be able to comprehend this readable text from editors with credibility. Dr Sudhir and Dr Manish also note couples who are affected by infertility may find it helpful in dealing with the problem and making decisions about their treatments.

Jayant G Mehta
Scientific Director
• Reproductive Care — London, UK
• Nawaloka Fertility Centre — Colombo, Sri Lanka
• Sub-Fertility, Queen's Hospital — Romford, UK
• Al-Mashari Hospital — Riyadh, Saudi Arabia

118, Cherrywood Lane
Morden. Surrey. SM4 4HB. UK.
Tel: +44 208 5422191
Mobile: +44 7954161488
Email: reproductivecare@gmail.c

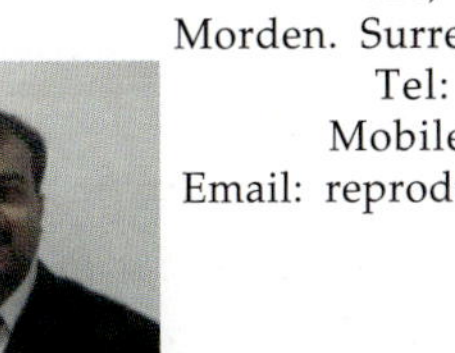

Dr Jayantbhai with Dr Manish Pandya

Preface

Infertility, in a broader sense is inability to conceive by a couple in spite of regular normal coitus by the couple involved. The time limit stamped as one year. Looking to the physiology of pregnancy both the partners are involved in this procedure.

In practice, females are considered to be the primary cause of it but the truth is different. Husband or a Male partner is responsible in 33% cases, and hence Male infertility Management is a key part in the practice of Total Infertility Management.

Numbers of books are written and read on Female problems and its managements on infertile couple. Problems of Male partners are equally important and should be thoroughly understood to manage it perfectly. Gone are the days when husband used to remain away when a case of sterility is being managed by an expert in the field. The time has changed now. Many pregnancies are not possible only because of the problems related to Male Partner. Change in the life style, tensions in professions and business, irregular and wrong habits, congenital factors and infections in childhood may interfere in sperm production and migration.

We have touched this untouched subject to give you the basics of such problems.

Reading this small booklet, confidence of managing male partner in your day to day practice will be doubled.

Make it a point to treat male partners at your own clinic routinely unless the need of some surgical rectification is needed.

We hope this book will enrich your knowledge in your day to day infertility practice.

Manish R Pandya
Sudhir R Shah

Acknowledgements

We are thankful to our idols and friends in this fraternity who encouraged penning this book.

Jaypee Brothers Medical Publishers for encouraging us and keeping full faith in us.

Mrs Jyoti Shah, Dr Nehal Manish Pandya MD DV and D (DERMATOLOGIST), better halves of the team of authors.

Numbers of our friends and colleagues who helped us in many ways.

Contents

CHAPTER 1

Sperm Production

We all know that this is the main component of male infertility if everything is normal and becomes the main source of infertility if everything is abnormal. So it totally depends on the knowledge of normal anatomy and molecular physiology of normal spermatozoa. In infertile male there is high incidence of numerical chromosomal aberration and abnormal sperm morphology.

WHAT WE WANT TO SEE IN NORMAL SPERMATOZOON?

This is very special cell that do not grow or divide.

Spermatozoon has usually head with paternal hereditary material DNA and big tail for motility (Fig. 1.1).

The specific difference from somatic cell is absent of large cytoplasm but endowed with large nucleus.

The posterior portion of the sperm head is covered by the post nuclear cap, which is a single membrane. The equatorial segment consist of an overlap of the acrosome and the post nuclear cap.

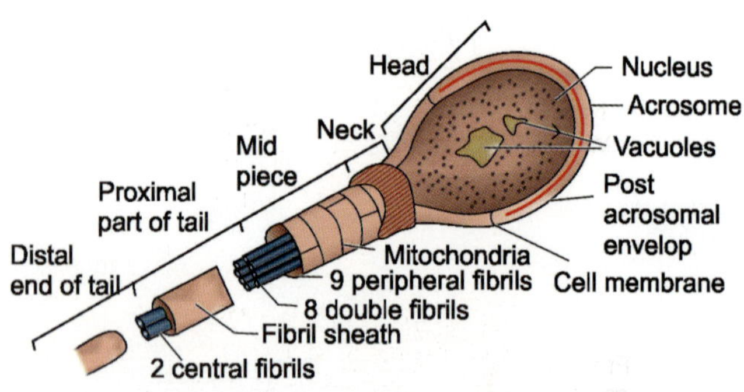

Fig. 1.1: Spermatozoa

The nucleus, constitutes 65 % of the head, is composed of DNA conjugated with protein.

Sperm nucleus can have incomplete condensation with apparent vacuoles. The genetic information carried by the spermatozoon is encoded and stored in the DNA molecules, which is made up of many nucleotides. The hereditary characteristic transmitted by the sperm nucleus include sex determination.

SPERM HEAD

Normal head is oval in shape 3 to 5 micrometer length and width is 2-3 micrometer (μm) (Fig. 1.2).

Head aberrations are as follows:
1. Shape and size
2. Large, small, tapering
3. Pyrifrom

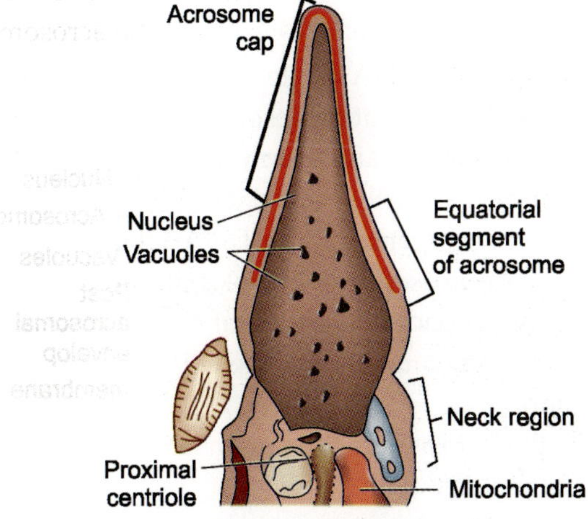

Fig. 1.2: Sperm head

4. Amorphous
5. Vacuolated
6. Double head.

Head is divided in two unequal parts

1. Acrosomal region
2. Postacrosome region

Head is usually flattened, ovoid and consists of nucleus only.

Acrosome is cap like and covers anterior 2/3 of head which arise from the golgi apparatus of the spermatid as it differentiate into spermatozoon (Fig. 1.3).

Hyaluronidase and proacrosin are in acrosome necessary for fertilization.

During fertilization of the egg, the enzyme rich contents of the acrosome are released at the time of acrosome reaction. During fusion of the outer acrosomal membrane with the Plasma membrane at multiple sites, the acrosomal enzymes are released.

The organization of DNA into loop domains is the only type of structural organization resolved so far and that is present in both somatic and sperm cells. DNA is coiled into nucleosomes, then further coiled into a 30 nm solenoid like fiber and then organized into DNA loop domains.

The mid piece possesses a cytoplasmic portion and a lipid reach mitochondrial sheath that consist of several spiral mitochondria, surrounding the axial filament in a helical fashion.

The mid piece provides the sperm with the energy necessary for motility (Fig. 1.4).

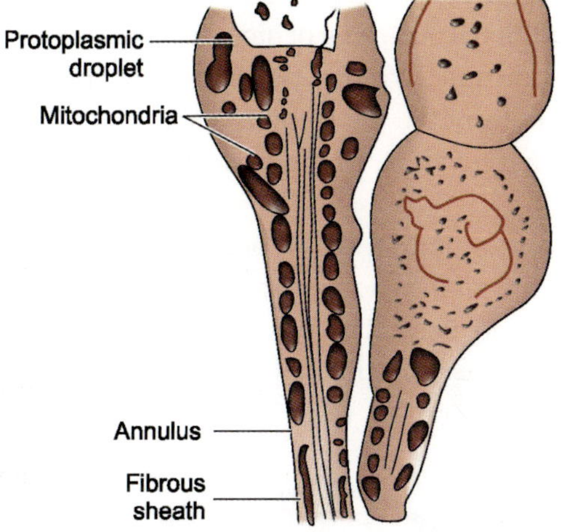

Fig. 1.3: L/s of mid piece

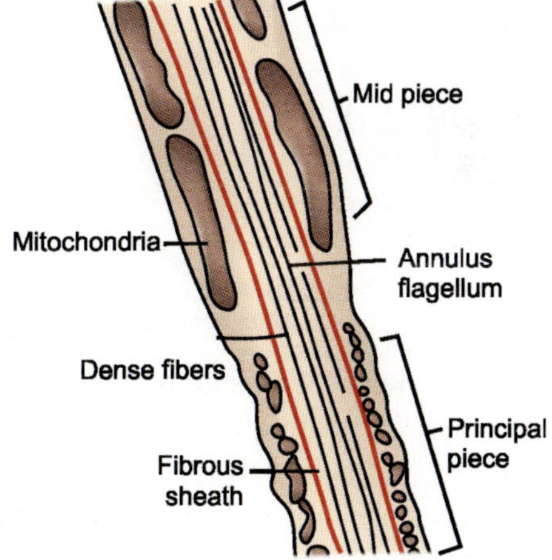

Fig. 1.4: L/s of mid piece and principal piece

The central axis core of eleven fibrils is surrounded by an additional outer ring of nine coarser fibrils. Individual mitochondrium is wrapped around these fibrils in a spiral manner to form the mitochondria sheath, which contains the enzyme involved in the oxidative metabolism of the sperm.

The mitochondrial sheath of the mid piece is relatively short, being slightly longer than the combined length of the head and neck. The principal piece (main piece) is the longest part of the tail, and provide most of the propellant machinery (Fig. 1.5).

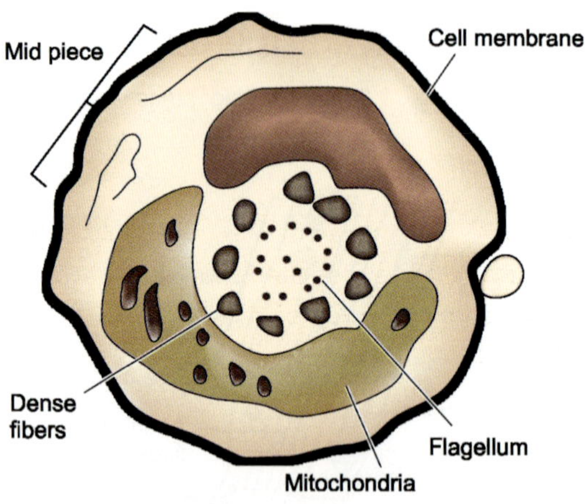

Fig. 1.5: Sperm tail

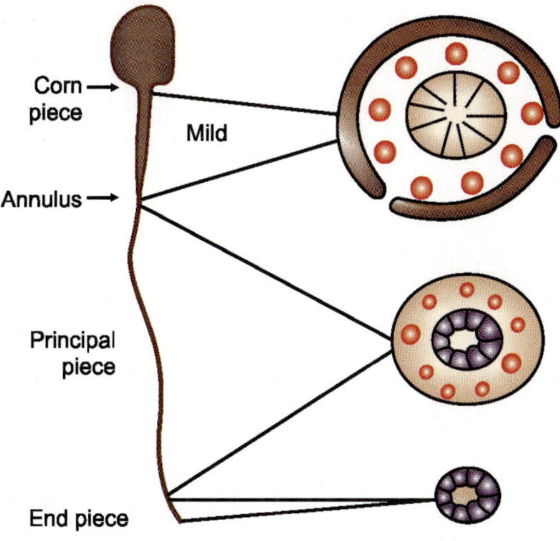

Fig. 1.6: Schematic representations of human spermatozoa

The coarse nine fibrils of the outer ring diminish in thickness and finally disappear leaving only the inner fibrils in the axial core for much of the length of the principal piece (Fig. 1.6).

CHAPTER 2

History and Investigation Taking

Infertility is now global problem and 10-12 % of couples are suffering form male infertility. This percentage rises upto 20 -25% when they conceive but are not able to reach completion and are not able to conceive for second time.

Infertility can be defined as the inability to conceive after a year of unprotected coitus in which intercourse has occurred in periovulatory period. Couple should be thoroughly evaluated for causes of infertility if they are not able to conceive after one year. This criterion should be of six months time for older couple.

It is very important to remember that infertility is just like bank joint account and must be operated with both signatures. So, physician have to go for evaluation of both partners to find out the cause. Evaluation of possibly infertile man demands through a gynecological review of his sexual partner in order to recognize any coexisting dysfunction.

HISTORY

Male infertility can be caused by many factors like:

1. Genetic
2. Neuroendocrine
3. Testicular
4. Urogenital.

A thorough examination of male with systemic evaluation is important in order to determine what therapeutic measure may be useful.

So many time personal history only is nonproductive. Physicians have to collect data on past marital status, family history, reproductive, developmental, past medical and surgical events, childhood disease, chronic disease, and most important occupation, environmental factors.

Marital History

1. Duration of infertility
2. Fertility of patients or his partner in previous marriage
3. Frequency of intercourse
4. Use of coital lubricants
5. Sexual potency
6. Sexual technique.

Childhood Disease

1. Cryptorchidism
2. Timing of puberty
3. Mumps in childhoods and not taken treatment.

Adult Illness

1. Mumps orchitis
2. Tuberculosis
3. Acute viral or febrile illness in past 3 months
4. Renal disease
5. Radiation therapy.

Surgery

1. Herniorrhaphy
2. Vasectomy
3. Retroperitoneal surgery.

Drugs

1. Alkalylating agents
2. Amebicide
3. Nitrofurantoin
4. Hormones
5. Alcohol and other drug abuse.

Occupational and Habits

1. Exposure to radiation and chemicals
2. Exposure to excessive heat, sauna baths
3. Wearing tight underwears, synthetic underwear.

SCROTAL TEMPERATURE

Several studies are conducted on effect of temperate on scrotum and physicians have found the littérateur that from scrotum if is insulated for long time there is detrimental effect on the sperm count and when motility and insulation is removed after some time, he gains his original motility and count.

This may be true for the patients who wear tight underclothes and physicians have seen that after changing the habit they improve a lot.

STRESS

In today's life stress is everywhere and if see surgical, occupational and psychological are of prime importance and studies have proved that this stress will decrease spermatogenesis and is most likely mediated by an adrenal-pituitary hypothalamic feedback mechanism.

In man, surgical stress and combat stress have shown to depress circulating testosterone levels.

ALCOHOL USE

Excessive use of alcohol can result in impotence or reduced fertility or increased progeny mortality.

Chronic alcoholism characterized by hepatitis, fatty liver, and cirrhosis reduce fertility indirectly by decreasing gonadotropins levels and directly by affecting the Leydig cells and reducing testosterone levels.

The androgen levels although low, may still be in normal range, but because of an increase in androgen binding globulin the levels of the free active forms of testosterone may be reduced.

Under such condition, if physician perform test of FSH and LH he will see elevation in hormonal levels.

This syndrome is characterized by testicular atrophy (biopsy reveal marked reduction in the germinal epithelium and peritubular fibrosis).

Other changes are gynecomastia, decreased growth of pubic, and body hairs.

70-80% cronic alcoholic males suffer from reduced libido, impotence and sterility.

When normal man consume large quantities of alcohol for as little as 5 days, a blunting of the episodic release and fall in the circulating level of testosterone occur and with increasing length of alcohol consumption this reduction continues.

CHAPTER 3

History of Male Infertility

Name

Age

Address

Date

General examination

Temp

Pulse

Bp

Weight

Height

Sings of virilization	normal	hypoandrogenism
Physical examination	normal	abnormal
Gynecomastia	absent	tanner stage

SEXUAL AND EJACULATORY FUNCTION

Erection

Ejaculation

Coital frequency

LOCAL EXAMINATION

Penis	normal	scar \ hypospadias / plaque\others
Testis	both palpable	nonpalpable
Site	normal	abnormal
Volume	left (ml)	right (ml)

Epididymis	normal	thickened \ tender \ cystic \ nonpalpable
Vasa differentia	normal	thicked \ nonpalpable
Scrotal swelling	none	hydrocele \ hernia
Varicocele	none	grade I\II\III \sub clinical
Inguinal examination	normal	lymphadenopathy \ infectious scar \ surgical scar \ hernia
Rectal examination		
Prostate	normal	soft swelling \ hard swelling / tender
Seminal vesicles	normal	palpable

PAST MEDICAL HISTORY (POSSIBLE INFLUENCE ON INFERTILITY)

History of medical treatment	no	DM \ TB \ RTI\ND
History of medical treatment	no	yes
High fever in past 6 months	no	yes
History of surgery	no	urethral stricture \ hypospadias
		prostatectomy \ bladder neck surgery
		vasectomy \ inguinal hernia
		hydrocelectomy \ sympathectomy

History of urinary tract infection	no	yes
History of STD	no	syphilis\gonorrhea\ chlamydia
History of epididymitis	no	yes
Mumps	no	yes\orchitis
History of varicocele treatment	no	yes
History of undesendent testis	no	yes\operation done

MISCELLANEOUS FACTOR

Environmental\occupational factor	no	yes heat\toxic factor
Excess alcohol consumption	no	yes
Drugs abuse	no	yes

SEXUAL AND EJACULATORY FUNCTION

Average frequency of vaginal

Intercourse/month	normal	inadequate
Erection	normal	inadequate
Ejaculation	normal	inadequate

GENERAL AND PHYSICAL EXAMINATION

Height (cm)

Weight (kg)

Blood pressure (mm Hg)		
General physical examination	normal	abnormal
Signs of virilization	normal	hypoandrogenism
Gynecomastia	absent	tanner stage

UROGENITAL EAXAMINATION

Penis	normal	scars plaques	hypospadias others
Testes	both palpable	nonpalpable	right left
Site	both normal	abnormal	right left
Volume (ml)	left right		
Epididymis	both normal	thickened tender cystic nonpalpable	
Vasa differentia	both normal	thickened nonpalpable	
Scrotal swelling	none	hydrocele hernia	
Varicocele	none	grade III grade II grade I sub clinical	
Inguinal examination	normal	lymphadenopathy Infection scars surgical scars hernia	

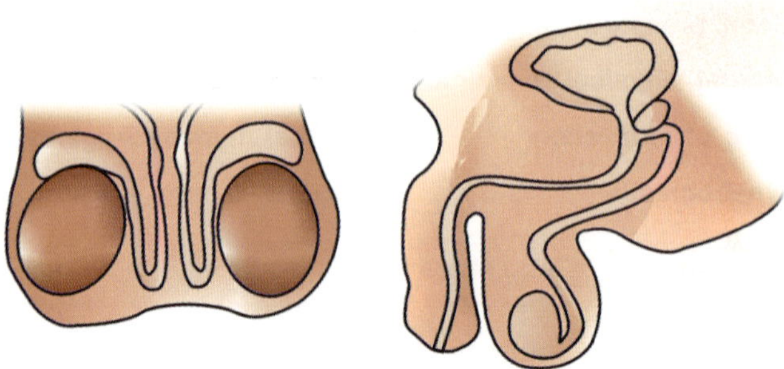

Fig. 3.1: Schematic diagram for history

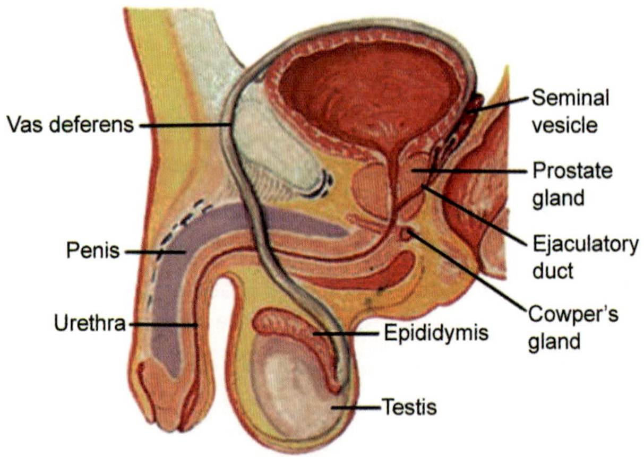

Fig. 3.2: Male genital organs

Rectal examination

Prostate	**normal**	**soft swelling**	**tender**
		hard swelling	**others**
Seminal vesicles	**normal**	**abnormal**	
(Contact thermography)			

Chapter 4

The Basic Semen Analysis

HISTORY OF SEMEN ANALYSIS

In 1677 van Leeuwenhoek's letter to The Royal Collage of London describing the discovery of the human spermatozoa by Johan Ham.

This was the starting note for sterile marriage and first attempt to establish diagnosis with aid of microscope.

In 19th century Lode was the first person to dilute semen sample and used hemocytometer for sperm count.

Belding was the first to through light on sperm morphology and added to this by Williams et al in *1934* by giving information on acrosome and vacuoles in sperm head.

Hotchkiss in 1941 published a basic grading system for sperm motility evaluation that was modified by MacLeod and Heim in 1945 to a system in which the motility and progressive activity were recorded separately.

American Fertility society have made standardization of a semen analysis in 1951.

Today physicians are following WHO manual published in 1980, 1987, 1992 and last 1999 for world standardizations of semen analysis.

As time advances and with advancement in ART techniques, physicians are also perform screening tests like, anti-sperm antibody such as MAR – Mixed antiglobulin reaction, leukocyte peroxidase test.

Sperm mucus penetration test is still very popular and used by many infertility specialists with periovulatory human cervical mucus or with human replacement like bovine mucus or hyaluronate. The sperm cervical mucus contact test, zona free hamster–ovum penetration test and hemizona assay test are some other techniques.

Recent advancement may include test like DNA status of the spermatozoa, the acrosome reaction test, ROS (The reactive oxygen species) activity of the spermatozoa especially leukocytes.

It is nowadays of utmost importance to have very good and skillful and perfect analysis of sperm in ART and ICSI.

BASIC SEMEN ANALYSIS

1. Background data
2. Physical analysis
3. Microscopic analysis
4. Additional procedure.

As per manual of WHO 1999, in present scenario of AIDS, Hepatitis B and Herpes, physicians have to take utmost care of own self before handling semen sample, must use protective gear like gloves, masks and spectacles.

Background Data

This is very important to know about the basic background data like:

- Time lapse between production and analysis
- Days of abstinence
- Type of container used.

The collection jar should be airtight and of good material which should not damage motility.

Physician must give good atmosphere to the person for collection of sample ideal is A/C room in close proximity to the laboratory and it is of utmost importance to do some special tests to be done before going for IVF.

When patient collects the sample near or at the laboratory a good relationship is created between patient and examiner and all questions are asked and will have rapid fire round for the questions.

Ideal method is masturbation and wide range of special condom are available for collection. Normal latex condoms are found to impair quality of sperm motility.

It is best for the patients to void urine before collection of sample and must wash hands with soap and clean glans with plain water before masturbation.

Physician must ask history of abstinence because it has profound effect on semen volume and sperm concentration. According to WHO manual, abstinence of 3-4 days is sufficient rather than 7 days which is too long.

For routine examination mentioning days are sufficient but for some special test and medical trials pathologist are now writing it is in hours of abstinence.

After production of sample it should be kept in CO_2 incubator at 37° temperature until it liquefies completely.

Physical Parameters

These include coagulation, liquefactions, viscosity, volume, color, odor and pH.

Coagulation is an important factor and it is only possible if it is produced within the vicinity of lab. Absent of coagulation is indicative of either absence of vas deferens and seminal vesicles and it also gives report of fructose negative as this is also produced by seminal plasma.

Semen is usually in liquid state at time of ejaculation and suddenly turns semisolid by action of enzyme protein kinase produced by seminal vesicle. Normal liquefactions occurs in 10-20 minutes and it is caused by proteolytic enzyme named fibrinolysis secreted by prostate and other two like fibrinogenase and aminopeptidase.

After whole sample liquefaction it appear homogeneous in composition and color. If patient has history of prostatitis, sample will take more than 20 minutes for liquefaction and sometime prostate is not functioning properly.

Viscosity is measured by pipette drop method and is normal if single drops are formed that are released within a distance of 20 mm from the point of the pipette. If threads are longer than 20 mm naturally viscosity is said to be increased and found to be related with abnormal prostatic function due to infection of prostate, seminal vesicle or whole genital tract.

Increase viscosity may be sometime cause of infertility. Normal volume is of 2-6 ml in standard 3-5 days of abstinence.

According to Hotchkiss the normal amount of volume is necessary for good buffering pool for acidic vagina to neutralized it.

Low volume may be caused first by wrong collection method or spillage and secondly physician has to give thought of obstruction due to previous infection or congenital absence of vas or seminal vesicle and very rarely it can also be due to retrograde ejaculation.

Normal color of semen is opaque and grayish and will chance to yellow as the day of abstinence increases.

There is typical odor of semen and its distinctive of its own. Physician can compare it with odor of chestnut or St John's bread tree. Usually cause of this odor is oxidation of the spermine secreted by the prostate, absence of odor is most commonly caused by infection.

pH of normal semen is ranging from 7.2 to 7.8.

pH of semen	*Indication*
> 8 →	Acute prostatitis, vesiculitis or epididymitis
< 7.2 →	Cronic infection
6.6 →	Obstruction of ejaculatory duct
< 7 →	Bilateral congenital absence of vas deferens

Microscopic Examination

All examination must be done under microscope at room temperature (ideal is body temperature, i.e. 37°C).

First examine under LPF low power filed and then HPF high power field.

Ideal method for examination size of drop of semen will depend on size of cover slip so the depth fluid and between the microscope slide and the cover slip is about 20 micrometer to allow maximum free movement of the spermatozoa.

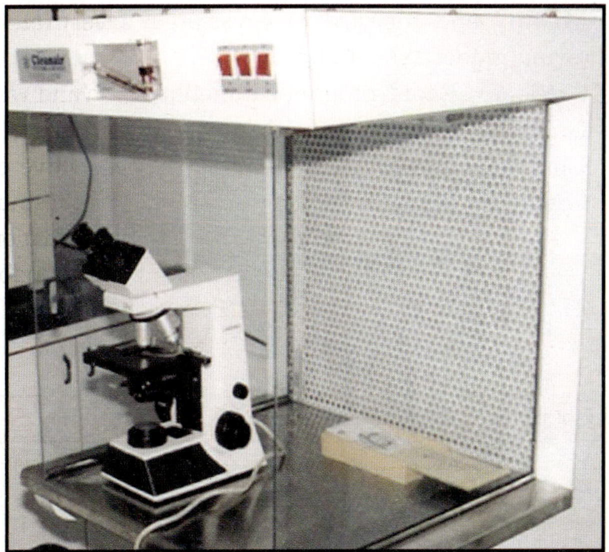

Fig. 4.1: Microscopic set up

First examine wet preparation under LPF to get impression of general appearance then HPF to have rough estimation of number of spermatozoa (Fig. 4.1).

Agglutinations are of two types—type 1 non-motile spermatozoa adhere to cells present in seminal plasma type 2 is specific agglutination caused by antisperm antibody which consists of motile spermatozoa clumps with only minimal involvement of other cell debris. Agglutination is termed as:

- Negative
- Occasional (+ –)
- Slight (+)
- Moderate (++)
- Severe (+++)

Motility and forward progression is classified in following grades (Fig. 4.2):

Grade a = Rapid progressive motility

Grade b = Slow or sluggish progressive motility

Grade c = Non-progressive motility

Grade d = Immotile.

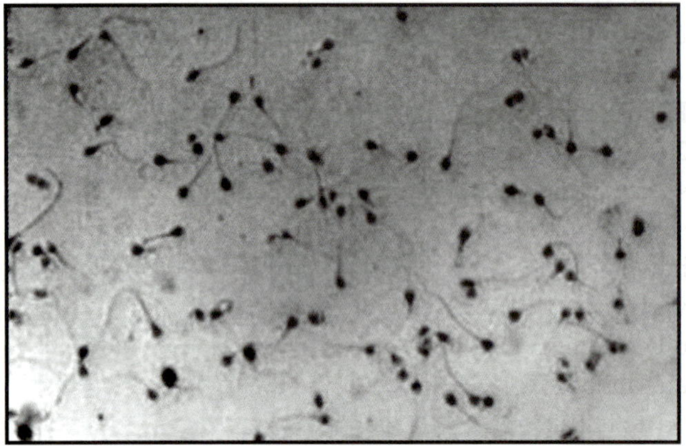

Fig. 4.2: Sperms

As it has been mention earlier in previous chapter poor motility and asthenoazoospermia can be caused by following factors:

- Wrong method of collection via use of condoms
- Use of lubricants
- An incomplete sample
- Long delay in transportation
- Exposure to extreme of temperature.

There are all the chances of artifact by using cold slides pipette, cold container, and wrong thickness of wet preparation.

For counting best is Makler chamber because it is possible to count directly on undiluted sample.

All laboratories are using 1:20 dilution made with white blood cell pipette and count is performed on a hemocytometer, diluting fluid consists of 5% sodium bicarbonate with 1% formalin.

In Neubauer chamber grid used for counting RBCs is used for number.

A latest reference table is given in WHO module and ESHRE manual indicating the number of blocks from the 25 to be included so that in all instances the number of spermatozoa will be more than 200.

A Tygerberg criterion for normal spermatozoa is one having and oval form with a smooth contour and a clearly visible and well defined acrosome with homogeneous light blue staining. The tail should be typically inserted without any abnormalities of the neck/mid piece region there should be no tail abnormalities and there should be no tail abnormalities and there should be no cytoplasmic residues at the neck region or on the tail (Table 4.1).

The size of a normal acrosome:

- Covers between 40-70% of anterior part of sperm head.
- With abnormal cytoplasmic droplets are present when larger than 50% of a normal sized sperm head.
- Measurement is 3.0-5.0 micrometer in length and 2.0-3.0 micrometer in width.

Mid piece should not be longer than 1.5 times a normal head and about 1 micrometer thick.

Tail should be about 45-50 micrometer long without any sharp bends.

Table 4.1: Classification of male's possible fertility potential

Author/semen parameter	*Infertile*	*Sub-fertile*	*Fertile*
Ombelet et al			
Concentration (10^6/ml)			34.00
Progressive motility (%)			45.0
Morphology (% normal)			10.0 (SC)
Guzick et al			
Concentration	< 13.5	13.5-48.0	> 48.0
Motility (% motile)	< 32.0	32.0-63.0	> 63.0
Morphology (% normal)	< 9.0	9.0-12.0	> 12.0 (SC)
Gunalp et al			
Concentration		9.0	
Progressive motility (%)		14.0	42
Morphology (% normal)		5.0	12.0 (SC)
Menkveld et al			
Motility (% motile)		20.0	45.0
Morphology (% normal)		21.0	31.0 (WHO)
Morphology (% normal)		3.0	4.0 (SC)
AI (% normal)		3.0	3.0
TZI (0-4)		2.09	1.64
Tygerberg hospital values			
Concentration (10^6/ml)	< 2.0	2.0 - 9.9	≥ 10.0
Motility (% motile)	< 10.0	10.0 - 29.0	≥ 30.0
Morphology (% normal)	< 5.0	5.0 - 14.0	≥ 15.0
Volume (ml)		<1.0 and > 6.0	1.0-6.0

AI = Acrosome index, TZI = Teratozoospermia index, SC = Strict Tygerberg criteria
WHO 1992 World Health Organization criteria

At least 200 spermatozoa should be evaluated in duplicate per slides.

Additional Tests

Teratozoospermia Index-TZI

It was introduced as an indication of the mean number of abnormalities per abnormal spermatozoon. So TZI value will be always between 1 and 4.

Latex MAR Test

In the test of latex MAR a drop of semen is placed on clean glass slide. Then add a drop of antiserum to human immunoglobulin (IgG) and a drop of the sensitized latex particle suspension. With the help of cover slip thoroughly mix all drops and examine under microscope by same cover slip after 10 minutes at room temperature.

Interpretation

Negative: no latex agglutination.
Doubtful: < 10 % motile sperm have latex particle bound.
Positive: 10-90% motile sperm shows latex particle bond.
Strongly positive: > 90 % motile sperm shows latex particle bonds.

In cases of positive MAR test blood and seminal plasma can be obtained for subsequent testing of antisperm antibody titer with the microagglutination and immobilization tests.

Leukocytes are usually associated with formation of ROS causing DNA damage and gives reduced rate of success with ART.

Most basic way to detect WBC in semen sample is direct observation under light microscope with aid of Papanicolaou's stain.

Origin of bacteriospermia might be because of normal colonization, contamination of sample or urogenital infection.

Male genital tract is usually bacteria free but male urethra may colonize many organisms.

Still there is much controversy regarding treatment with antibiotics for leukocytospermia but physician can use doxycycline, erythromycin and trimethoprim in combination with sulfamethoxazole and post-treatment result will be improvement in sperm quality.

Sperm Vital Staining Test

A drop of semen is placed on a spot plate and mixed with one drop of 1% aqueous eosin Y solution after 15 seconds two drops of 10% aqueous nigrosin solution are added and mixed thoroughly → put one drop of mixture on slide for examination under oil immersion → red cells or any sperm cells not totally white are regarded as dead, and the results are expressed as the percentage of live (white) sperm.

The performance of a vital stain technique is an important tool to distinguish between live but motionless and dead spermatozoa.

Necrozoospermia is condition where all spermatozoa are found to be dead by vital staining.

AZOOSPERMIA

When examination of semen sample shows no spermatozoa, it is azoospermia.

Second examination usually done after centrifuging of sample and supernatant is carefully examined for presence of any spermatozoa.

If spermatozoa present = cryptozoospermia or oligoazoospermia, i.e. $< 1 \times 10^6$ spermatozoa/ml.

CASA (Computerized Assisted Sperm Morphology Analysis)

Williams and Sevage said "in the microscopic study of spermatozoa the morphology of sperm head constitute the greatest single source of information as to the fitness of these cells for reproduction".

Recently the controversy on morphology assessment has been reviewed through claims that the application of

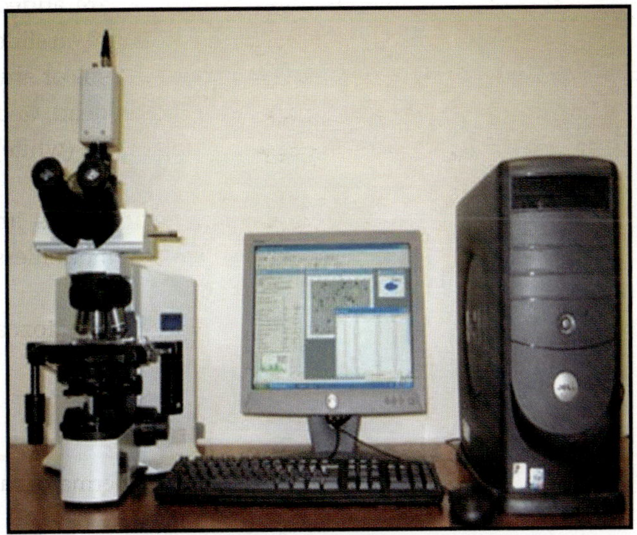

Fig. 4.3: CASA

strict criteria for normality would give better results in terms of reproducibility, clinical accuracy and predictive power than the more liberal criteria described by WHO.

In order to evaluate the correctness of this assumption, and also to assess the accuracy of the fully automatic computerized assisted systems for sperm morphology (CASA), multicenteric study was performed and results shows CASA systems matched closely in terms of reproducibility and correspondence with the average results of all centers (Fig. 4.3).

Chapter 5

Male Factor—Infertility and Ejaculatory Duct

Male – storehouse of sperm—which unites with ovum of female and creates a totally unique and genetically irreplaceable, incompatible one of its own - human life—a wonderful amazing process (Fig. 5.1).

Infertility is not a just woman's problem but it is couple's problem.

Male factors are sometimes the main cause of infertility; otherwise it is 33% cause of infertility in total.

Husband and wife should be interviewed, examined and investigated simultaneously.

Normal male in one ejaculate releases 120-600 million sperm at each time; statistically male is manufacturer of 40000000000 sperms in lifetime.

Why husband semen report is not found many a times…

Practically it is not so but unless we write requisition form of HSE (Husband semen examination) but condition for not undergoing to laboratory are:

1. Husband is not coming with wife.
2. Abstinence is not proper (minimum it should be above five days).
3. Husband is not able to give semen in laboratory.
4. Husband is resisting and says I am okay because I can perform well.
5. Mother-in-law says my son is okay and he will not under go any investigation.
6. Psychological disturbances while collecting sample and not able to ejaculate or no erection at all.
7. Collection at home and taking in dicey of scooter.
8. Not proper time for reaching to laboratory.

9. Very rarely but it may happen that husband knows regarding his status of azoospermia and resists for investigation—very common in second marriage after divorce for infertility.
10. Male dominant society.

Male factor of infertility are around the male genital organ mostly or we have to search for endocrinopathy and rarely we have to go for karyotype for the same.

LOCAL FACTORS

Why we are Insisting for Local Factor?

This is most common and easily identifiable cause and it will serve your examination capability as consultant.

Now with this chapter we insist on male partner examination as routine in infertility practice because it will serve so many purposes of yours and easily identifiable causes corrected immediately.

Till today our branch of obstetrics and gynecology is mostly managed by female gynecologists and easy argument is we are not examining male and practically speaking it is true also but if you see mostly female gynecologist have male partner and usually he will be of medicine speciality, then take help of him for better outcome of infertility.

If female dermatologist examines male for STD VD sexual problems then why not female gynecology not doing so?

If we look at the factors, causing male infertility, they are:

1. The inability to produce number of healthy sperms.

2. Inability to deliver sperms into vagina, e.g. impotence, an ejaculate, retrograde ejaculation.
3. Others are:
   - Ejaculatory dysfunction
   - Vericocele
   - Sepsis
   - Male accessory gland inflammation
   - Congenital factor
   - Acquired causes
   - Testicular cancer.

In the recent years number of modalities in the treatment have emerged, especially for impotence, e.g. penile implant, sildenafil ejaculation—Vibrator, electroejaculation.

Psychological treatment by counseling sitting with psychotherapist for disturbed male to feel him more confident of himself.

IUI – is nowadays, time tested and treatment from gynecology in full association with andrology lab give very good useful sample of semen in case of oligospermia.

Better laboratory facility will give good understanding of male sperm and its physiology very well.

ART is an art of todays science in lovely hands of gynecologists by which gynecologists can give new life to couple of infertility. Causes of male infertility can be overcome by procedure like ICSI (Intracytoplasmic sperm injection). Macho man not able to produce even single sperm can satisfy his ego and become father of his own child by testicular aspiration.

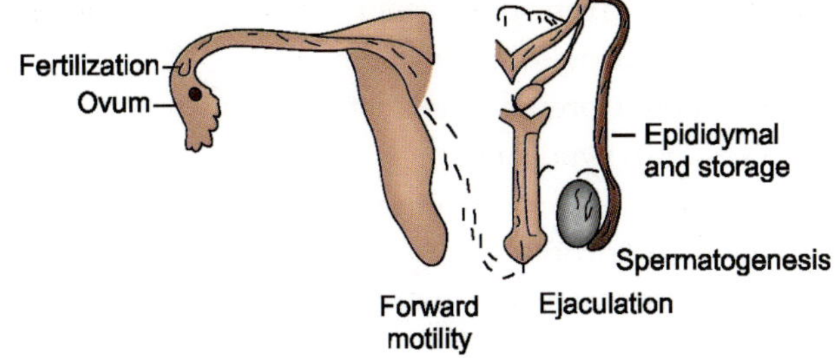

Fig. 5.1: Normal fertilization

CAUSES OF MALE INFERTILITY

Causes of male infertility are divided into following categories:

1. Disorder of spermatogenesis
2. Production disorder
3. Transportation disorder
4. Erectile dysfunction (procreation)
5. Ejaculatory dysfunction
6. Meeting problem (couple disorder)

DISORDER OF SPERMATOGENESIS

Idiopathic Oligoazoospermia or Azoospermia

Congenital or developmental disorder:

1. Vericocele
2. Cryptorchidism
3. Klinefelter's syndrome

4. Myotonic dystrophy
5. Sertoli cell only syndrome
6. Functional prepubertal castrate syndrome
7. Noonan's syndrome
8. Polyglandular autoimmune disease
9. Down syndrome
10. Complex genetic syndrome.

Acquired Disorder

1. Orchitis
2. Drugs – cytotoxic drugs, sulphasalazine, alcohol, marijuana, ketoconazole, cyclosporine, flutamide, histamine receptor antagonist
3. Irradiation
4. Hyperthermic injuries
5. Spinal cord injury
6. Environmental toxines (e.g. DBCP)
7. Surgical or traumatic castration/physical trauma.

Systemic Disorder

1. Hepatic cirrhosis
2. Chronic renal failure
3. Malignancy, e.g. Hodgkin's disease, testicular carcinoma
4. Vasculities (Periarterits)
5. Infiltrative disease (Amyloidosis)
6. Sickle cell disease.

PRODUCTION DISORDER (SECONDARY HYPOGONADISM)

Congenital or Developmental Disorder

1. Hypogonadotropic eunuchoidism (Kallamann's syndrome)
2. Hematocromatosis
3. Complex genetic syndrome.

Acquired Disorder

1. Hypopituitarism (destructive or infiltrative pituitary disease
2. Hyperprolactinemia
3. Androgen excess (congenital adrenal hyperplasia, androgen secreting tumors)
4. Estrogen excess or progestogens
5. Opiate like other active drugs.

Systemic Disorder

1. Glucocorticoid excess (Cushing's syndrome)
2. Nutritional deficiency (e.g. malnutrition, anorexia nervosa)
3. Acute and chronic stress or illness
4. Massive obesity.

Androgen Resistance Syndrome

1. Reifenstein's syndrome
2. Idiopathic oligoazoospermia or azospermia
3. 5α-reductase deficiency
4. Celiac disease.

DISORDER OF SPERM TRANSPORT AND ACCESSORY GLAND FUNCTION

Ductal Obstruction

1. Congenital defects of vas, seminal vesicle or epididymis (e.g. cystic fibrosis)
2. Young's syndrome
3. Mullerian duct cyst
4. Vasectomy
5. Post-infection obstruction of epididymis, seminal vesicle or vas.

Impaired Sympathetic Innervations of Ducts

1. Spinal cord disease
2. Sympathectomy or sympatholytic drugs
3. Retroperitoneal lymphadenectomy
4. Vasovasostomy.

Epididymal and Accessory Gland Dysfunction

1. Androgen deficiency or resistance
2. Hyperthermic injury
3. Genital tract infection.

CAUSES OF ERECTILE DYSFUNCTION

Central Nervous System Disorder

1. Psychiatric disturbance
2. Emotional stress or performance anxiety
3. Depression
4. Major psychiatric illness.

Chronic Medical Illness

1. Cardiac, respiratory, renal or liver disease
2. Malignancy
3. CNS active antihypertensive
4. Anti-depressants
5. Anti-psychotics
6. Sedative-hypnotics
7. Alcohol.

Endocrine Disorder

1. Androgen deficiency or resistance
2. Hyperprolactinemia
3. Thyroid disease.

CNS Disease

Temporal lobe or limbic system disorder.

Spinal Cord Disease

1. Spinal cord injury
2. Multiple sclerosis
3. Transverse myelitis
4. Tumors
5. Vascular compromise
6. Epidural abscess
7. Spinal stenosis or spina bifida
8. Syphilis.

Autonomic Nervous System Dysfunction

1. Pelvic surgery
2. Diabetic autonomic neuropathy

3. Other peripheral neuropathy
4. Drugs affecting peripheral erectile response
5. Anticholinergic drugs
6. Antidepressants
7. Alpha-adrenergic antagonists
8. Antihistamines
9. Antihypertensive drugs
10. Sympathomimetic agents
11. Alpha-adrenergic agonists.

Vascular Disease

1. Distal aortic disease
2. Penile arterial disease (e.g. diabetes)
3. Venous incompetence.

Penile Abnormalities

1. Peyronie's disease or chordae
2. Micropenis
3. Penile trauma
4. Priapism.

DISORDER OF EJACULATION

Premature or Retarded Ejaculation

Retrograde Ejaculation

Bladder Neck Surgery

1. Prostatectomy
2. Bladder neck incision
3. Y-V ureterocystoplasty.

Sympathetic Nervous Dysfunction

1. Autonomic neuropathy (e.g. diabetes)
2. Sympatholytic drugs or sympathectomy
3. Retroperitoneal or abdominal pelvic surgery
4. Spinal cord injury.

Retrograde Ejaculation

1. Androgen deficiency or resistance
2. Sympathetic nervous system dysfunction
3. Urethral abnormalities (e.g. stricture, hypospadias, epispadias).

COITAL DISORDER AND DISORDER OF SPERM TRANSPORT

Coital Disorder

1. Infrequent intercourse
2. Excessive intercourse or masturbation
3. Poor timing in relationship to ovulation
4. Premature withdrawal.

Disorder of Sperm Functions

1. Sperm toxic lubricants
2. Sperm dysmotility
3. Idiopathic asthenospermia
4. Immotile cilia syndrome (Kartagener's syndrome)
5. Protein carboxylmethylase deficiency
6. Immunologic (antisperm antibodies)
7. Idiopathic polyazoospermia

CHAPTER 5-A

WHAT IS A NORMAL EJACULATION?

The normal ejaculatory respond consists of well timed neuromuscular events that result in the expulsion of semen from urethra.

A decrease or absence of fertility potential in the nerves or the muscle related to this phenomenon is the result of anatomical abnormalities of the ejaculatory organs.

Ejaculatory dysfunction is uncommon and account for 2%.

(Dublin L 1971—etiological factor in 1294 cases of male infertility):

Rainbow of clinical causes are:

1. Anejaculation
2. Retrograde ejaculation
3. Premature ejaculation
4. Ejaculatory duct obstruction.

Anejaculation and ejaculatory dysfunction are terms used to describe male infertility as inability to have ejaculation by neurological disease, traumatic injury or as complication of surgery.

For diagnosis of proper causes, understanding of physiology of ejaculation and etiology of each disorder enable physician to select appropriate treatment.

PHYSIOLOGY OF EJACULATION

Ejaculatory reflex is to coordinate events initiated by cerebral integration of visual, auditory, tactile and olfactory stimuli modulated by psychosocial cognitive processing.

Tactile stimuli to the afferent receptors on the glans penis travel through the pudendal nerve from the glans to the brain. The efferent neuronal pathways arise from thoracolumbar spinal level (T 10-L2) and travel through the sympathetic chain ganglia to the hypogastric plexus, then through the pelvis (as the hypogastric nerve) and terminate as postganglionic fibers on the prostate, vas deference, and seminal vesicles.

Sympathetic stimulation causes a concerted sequence of events-closure of the bladder neck prevents retrograde ejaculation; and contraction of the prostatic musculature, ampulla of the vas deference and seminal vesicle cause emission of the semen and seminal fluid into the prostatic urethra.

As the urogenital diaphragm opens, propulsion of semen through the urethra is then maintained by rhythmic contraction of the bulbocavernosus, ischiocavernosus and the pelvic floor muscles under the somatic motor control of the pudendal nerve (S2-S4).

Numerous short adrenergic fibers are located throughout the wall of the vas deference.

Recently we have seen new role of NO (Nitrus oxide) in male infertility as high concentration of NO is found in epididymis, vas deference and seminal vesicle.

ETIOLOGY OF EJACULATORY DYSFUNCTION

Most of the ejaculatory dysfunctions are traumatic or iatrogenic.

ANEJACULATION

Traumatic Causes

1. Spinal cord injury
2. Trauma to posterior urethra.

Iatrogenic

1. Retroperitoneal lymph node dissection
2. Aortic aneurysectomy (operation of aortic aneurysm)
3. Colorectal surgery
4. Sympathectomy.

Pharmacological

1. Antihypertensive
2. Antipsychotics
3. Antidipressant
4. Others (Alcohol, baclofen).

Metabolic and Systemic Disease

1. Diabetes mellitus
2. Multiple sclerosis
3. Bone marrow transplant.

Psychological

1. Retarded ejaculation.

Idiopathic

Traumatic

Spinal cord injuries (SCI) may cause anejaculation in 90-95 % sufferers.

Usually these male population is young with average age of 25-30 years and mostly suffered by vehicular or some accident followed by spinal injury and lead to anejaculation.

SCI make patients suffer from variety of sexual function and abnormalities depending on level of injury at cord site.

Men with complete upper motor neuron lesion rarely ejaculate but most of them are capable of sufficient erection for intercourse to satisfy spouse.

Men with incomplete upper motor neuron disease mostly retain capability of ejaculation.

Men with complete lower motor neuron decrease can ejaculate and have erection while incomplete lower motor neuron lesion can maintain erection but only half can achieve ejaculation.

In category of SCI anejaculation, only few percentage; can go for pregnancy mostly they have to take help of ART specialist and have go for test tube (IVF).

Iatrogenic

Surgical injury to sympathetic nerves may result in retrograde ejaculation.

Retroperitoneal lymph node dissection, incases of non-seminiferous testicular tumors, can sometime causes anejaculation by accidental injury to sympathetic trunk or sometimes more peripheral postganglionic sympathetic fibers disrupting the ejaculatory mechanism.

Abdominal aorta aneurysm surgery like aneurysmectomy can cause retrograde ejaculation.

Anterior resection for colonic surgery sometimes causes injury to anterior hypogastric plexus and can cause ejaculatory disturbance.

TURP (Transurethral resection of prostate) can cause vesicle neck incompetence and retrograde ejaculation incidence upto 90%.

If husband wants to have antegrade ejaculation he has to go for medical therapy rather than to go for surgery and can take medicine like Terazocin, Finasteride.

Sometimes undiagnosed urethral stricture can cause retrograde ejaculation.

Surgery like Y-V urethroplasty of the vesicle neck, for high outflow, tract resistance and ureterovesical reflux in childhood must be investigated for presence of retrograde ejaculation because they may now be in reproductive age group in present scenario.

Congenital

Congenital absence of vas and seminal vesicle is most common cause of azoospermia when we see low volume ejaculate (<1 ml) and usually this semen is acidic.

Rare circumstances are congenital mullerian duct cyst.

Childhood surgery for bladder extrophy, epispadias.

Sometimes urethral valves or myelodysplasia can cause anejaculation or retrograde ejaculation.

Pharmacological

Nowadays, in era of high tension which reflects in hypertension and runs towards success, sometimes causes severe depression and those to males have to go for consultation and take medicine for antihypertension and antidepressant.

Agents associated with impaired ejaculation:

1. Alcohol
2. Amitryptyline
3. Baclofen
4. Bethanidine
5. Chlordiazepoxide
6. Chlorimipramine
7. Chlorpromazine
8. Chlorprothixene
9. Clomipramine
10. EPAC (Epsilone Animo Caproic acid)
11. Guanethidine sulfate
12. Haloperidol
13. Hexamethionin
14. Imipramine hydrochloride
15. Methadone
16. Naproxen
17. Pargyline
18. Perphenazine
19. Phenelzine sulfate
20. Phenoxybenzamine hydrochloride
21. Phenotamine
22. Prazosin hydrochloride
23. Reserpine
24. Thaizides
25. Thioridazine
26. Trifluoperazine hydrochloride.

Agents used to achieve seminal emission and/or antegrade ejaculation:

1. Bromopheniramine meleate
2. Chlorpheniramine
3. Ephedrine sulfate
4. Imipramine hydrochloride
5. Phenylpropanolamine
6. Pseudoephedrine hydrochloride

While prescribing these drugs to the patients we have to be careful of their sexual activity.

Metabolic and Systemic Disease

Patients with Diabetes mellitus usually suffer from autonomic neuropathy with erectile dysfunction, and some of them also suffer from retrograde ejaculation. This problem is very common in young patients with juvenile onset DM.

Multiple sclerosis, a demylenating disease, may be associated with anejaculatation or premature ejaculation.

Inflammatory

Urogenital inflammation involving the ejaculation ducts may cause partial or complete obstruction.

Chronic prostatitis have shown ejaculatory duct obstruction, possibly associated with premature ejaculation.

Prolonged catheterization may induce an inflammatory reaction that can obstruct the orifice of the ejaculatory ducts at the level of verumontanum.

Other inflammatory lesion, such as advanced tuberculosis and gonococcal urethritis may be associated with bilateral vassal and epididymal scarring.

Psychological

Numerous psychological conditions may be associated with functional disorder of ejaculation.

Some of them are as follows:

1. Subconscious sadistic feeling towards partner
2. Performance anxiety
3. Fear of sexually transmitted disease
4. Illicit situation where the need to perform quickly
5. Unresolved marital problem
6. Olfactory improper sensation
7. Disfigurement of spouse
8. Uncomfortable position.

Psychodynamic bases of ejaculatory incompetence (retarded ejaculation):

1. Fear of unwanted pregnancy
2. Consideration of religious orthodoxy
3. Lack of sexual desire
4. Fear of congenital anomaly in potential offspring
5. Distorted body image.

Idiopathic

May be of myogenic or neurogenic origin and should be in back of mind when volume of an ejaculate is small and acidic (very few sperm seen microscopically).

Presence of sperm in catheterized post-ejaculatory urine sample can diagnose this condition.

Characteristically nocturnal emissions is present in these cases and indicate that ejaculatory reflex is present and problem is psychological.

Diagnosis

Ejaculatory dysfunction disorder is not difficult to diagnose if one is keen to see the existence of the differential.

So many times etiologies can provide important sources of information in this disorder.

ANEJACULATION

Anejaculation is complete absence of antegrade ejaculation.

This category of patients may experience sometime normal or decrease orgasm with contraction but nothing to ejaculate.

Normally what ever teacher had taught us regarding history taking will solve the problem because history is mostly evident in all types of cases.

If semen analysis is not done in these cases as there is no ejaculate, post-orgasm urine analysis shows non viscous there is fructose negative sperm negative sample.

RETROGRADE EJACULATION

Retrograde ejaculation is established when post-intercourse or masturbation urine analysis shows spermatozoa under microscopic vision.

Ideally for all retrograde ejaculate sample, whole content of bladder is centrifuged and then semen sample (sediments) again suspended in 1 ml of media before microscopic examination should be and motility parameters.

PREMATURE EJACULATION

According to MASTERS and JOHNSON premature ejaculation is the condition where there is inability to control or sustain ejaculation for a sufficient length of time during intravaginal containment to satisfy female in at least 50% of coital events.

In classical case this happens before or immediately upon vaginal penetration and typically by emission and ejaculation is followed by loss of erection.

In milder variety chief complaint of patients will be like inadequate intravaginal endurance prior to ejaculation and usually it is of male concern only.

This is dual history diagnosis after consultation of both partners.

EJACULATORY DUCT OBSTRUCTION

Mostly this diagnosis is evidence based as we have to depend on laboratory findings in cases where we see small ejaculate, azospermia and fructose negative sample.

Difficulty arises in diagnosis when there is unilateral or partial block or sometimes only functional blocks may give false report form normal site.

Local examination can diagnose thick palpable cord. TRUS (Transrectal sonography) sometimes may show cyst.

Suspicion of ejaculatory duct obstruction should arise when physician sees normal report of gonadotropins with normal size testis with small volume ejaculate with fructose absent and physician must investigate this type of patients and eventually we achieve good report with correction of problem.

TRUS may show enlargement of seminal vesicle or distension of intraprostatic ejaculatory ducts.

Vasography is radiological demonstration of blockage but we believe that it should be planned before surgical repair scheduled.

Alternative diagnostic modality is chromopertubation like method in which (vas deferens) instillation of indigo carmine dye for followed by examination of catheterized urine is presence of dye in it but this methods will not elicit the exact site of blockage.

Newer diagnostic technique in form of MRI is equivocal important for very good visualization of seminal vesicle and prostate but with TRUS we get the same results.

TREATMENT

Therapeutic evaluation and causal treatment is given according to etiology.

MEDICATION

As we have already mentioned that numerous pharmacological drugs ejaculatory dysfunction can cause, after proper sorting of the drug either switch over to another molecule or it may require stoppage of drug also.

Routinely a normal treatment in patients with retrograde ejaculation will be to advise patients to do intercourse with full bladder and they will ejaculate antegrade.

In patients without neurological or bladder neck scarring form of ejaculatory dysfunction will be benefited with sympathomimetic drugs—sometimes single drug is not sufficient and we have to give combination of drugs also.

Much success will be seen in patients with retroperitoneal lymph node dissection. Results show conversion of retrograde to antegrade ejaculation, increase in sperm counts in previously low sperm density in patients with ejaculatory failure.

Alpha-adrenergic sympathomimetic agents act through increased closure pressure at the internal urinary sphincter via release of norepinephrine from the terminal nerve endings and stimulation of adrenergic receptor sites.

Drugs like imipramine hydrochloride, a tricyclic antidepressant, blocks their uptake of norepinephrine at nerve terminals, potentiating the adrenergic activity.

Imipramine possesses anticholinergic and direct smooth muscle relaxant property and should be used in patients with some neurological, gastrointestinal and cardiac disease.

In patients with anejaculation, physician can use injectable (hCG) human chorionic gonadotropins and it will lead to nocturnal emission, which can be collected in non-spermicidal condom, and used for AIH.

People had tried low dose of phenothiazines for use in premature ejaculation and found very good result in form of satisfaction to both patient as well as partner because it has got property of anxiolitic and mood elevation.

Phenoxybenzamine can be used in patients who do not want to procreate and just want to delay ejaculation.

CHEMICAL EJACULATION

Word sounds like not hear about this type of ejaculation until one sees only ejaculation of semen from urethra not the chemical ha-ha... ha...

Exactly this is very new and very old method of getting ejaculation from previously spinal cord injured man.

Guttmann first reported use of intrathecal injection of neostigmine in patients with spinal cord injury; drug, an inhibitor of acetylcholine esterase has been found to reduce spasticity and to heighten sexual function in some patients.

60 % of patients found to be erectile for several hours and many found dribbling ejaculation of semen for couple of days with or without accompanying erection. The ejaculation occurs either antegrade or retrograde depending on status of bladder neck function.

The best result is seen with intrathecal injection of neostigmine in patients with incomplete lesion of cord while least success will be seen in patients with lesion from T10 to L4, i.e. origin of sympathetic outflow responsible for emission.

You will be surprised that till today why we are not trying to use this wonderful drug in our patients to get fantastic results. Because of its tremendous side effects like autonomic dysreflexia, transient loss of bowel and bladder function, muscular weakness. Serious hypertensive crisis may require continuous cardiac monitoring and nitroprusside—a vasodilator and sometime hospitalization.

Chappell had used subcutaneous Physostigmine as it crosses blood-brain barrier. It does not require intrathecal administration.

Use of both drugs is abandoned because of its side effects.

So one should think of new chemical use for chemical ejaculation.

Yes at present, physicians are using intracavernous injection of agents like Papaverine and Phentolamine or Prostaglandin E1 for the treatment of premature ejaculation.

In patients on psychological therapy and with psychological impotence on physicians are finding very good results with intracavernous injection but still it will require more number of patients for the study.

PSYCHOLOGICAL THERAPY

Premature ejaculation rarely affects fertility unless it occurs before vaginal penetration; sometime we collect even permute ejaculate and use it for AIH. Standard method of management in this type of case requires more of counseling and sex therapy.

Prime motto of counseling is to increase pre ejaculatory time.

Physicians try 'squeeze technique' in which patients has to compress penis before sensation of ejaculation; and second is to avoid sexual thought while intercourse; sometime use of local anesthetic agents like xylocaine at urethra.

For bladder neck, scarring surgical correction will solve problem of retrograde ejaculation.

Congenital cystic lesion of the ejaculatory ducts have been managed by Transurethral unroofing or resection of the verumontanum to relieve obstruction.

If patients present with both, ejaculatory duct as well as epididymal obstruction, surgical correction can be done in form of transurethral resection of the ejaculatory duct and vasoepididymostomy.

Microsurgical repair of vassal obstruction is associated with higher pregnancy rates.

Challenging surgery is when we have to go for vasoepididymal anastomosis as epididymis has little or no muscular support of its delicate mucosa.

The epididymides have an important role in acquisition of sperm motility and fertilizing capacity and it is true that greater length of exposure of sperm in epididymis greater the chances of fertility.

Microsurgical sperms combined with ART is nowadays trends in case of vas block because of tuberculosis or even after failed vasoepididymal anastomosis.

Microepididymal sperm aspiration (MESA) is boon to the group of patient with congenital absence of vas.

PENILE VIBRATORY STIMULATION

If reader looks at the history of vibro, stimulator has been used for the male who are neurologically normal but there is anejaculation.

Normally it is a sympathetic event of the efferent neuronal pathways arising from spinal level T10 to L2.

This is very useful technique for the patients with spinal cord injury because penile vibratory stimulation mandates an intact neurotical and anatomical apparatus below the level of neurological deficit.

Most of the time physician can get successful ejaculation if there is active central and peripheral neuroaxis below the T10 level.

In patients with retroperitoneal lymphadectomy, penile vibrostimulation is not useful because sympathetic pathways are surgically interrupted.

First, physician have to evacuate the bladder before vibrostimulation either in supine or relaxed sitting position. If this is a case of retrograde ejaculation then we have to fill bladder with 30 ml of buffer media probably with Ham f10 and leave indwelling catheter before stimulation.

The tip of the vibrator is placed on the undersurface of the glans penis, compressed lightly, and moved from side to side.

When you reach the trigger point you wills see sudden enhancement of tumescence or an increase in abdominal or lower extremity spasticity.

When the threshold level of activation is reached, the ejaculatory sequence is initiated and there is final increase in corporeal tumescence and rigidity often noted.

Although the ejaculatory and erectile spinal reflexes are distinct but there is some neural communication does exist to explain the erectile augmentation that occurs just before ejaculation.

Semen proper through the urethra is collected in sterile container and sent to laboratory for ICSI and future preservation for next cycle.

The main side effect of vibratory stimulation is autonomic dysreflexia but it wanes off shortly after removing stimulator.

TRANSRECTAL ELECTROEJACULATION

Rectal electroejaculation is in veterinary science and very old in practice.

People are trying different modes of stimulation like with finger electrode probe stimulation.

Most common indication for this is spinal cord injury and usually in patients with paraplegia, is with retroperitoneal lymphadectomy.

Less commonly, this can be used in cases of myelodysplasia, diabetic neuropathy, multiple sclerosis.

In this technique, retrograde ejaculation occurs most frequently. So physician has to fill the bladder with sufficient amount of buffer media to collect the viable sperms.

Different sizes of probes are available for stimulation at level of peri-prostatic plexus in order to stimulate neuronal activity for ejaculation.

Physician may encounter rectal mucosa, minor burns and some times rectal perforation, which might require colostomy.

SPERM ENRICHMENT

Best way to get good quality sperms after retrograde ejaculation is bladder enrichment with buffer media to make urine at least 200-300 mosm/L; usually urine is 366 msom/L and at this pH, sperm loses its motility.

Physician can advice patient to take more sodium bicarbonate or acetazolamide for several days.

Sperm cryopreservation is done prior to surgical procedures for testicular carcinoma or retroperitoneal lymph node dissection.

Retrograde ejaculate are preserved for future ICSI procedure.

Post thaw sample use of Pentoxifylline and PAF (platelets activating factor) enhance the motility.

Advancement in sperm retrieving and processing techniques will make ART very easy for ejaculatory dysfunctional males.

Chapter 6

Medical Approach for Male Infertility

Truly, this is very challenging topic and as a physician we know that not much of treatment can be offered to male compared to female.

First we have to understand about the basics of spermatogenesis.

Normal spermatogenesis will require adequate testicular stimulation.

Pulsatile secretion of LHRH (Lutenizing hormone releasing hormone) by hypothalamus induces pulsatile release of LH (Lutenizing hormone), which sequentially causes pulsatile release of testosterone by Leydig cell.

Extreme high concentration of testosterone is found in interstitial fluid surrounding the tubule.

Hypogonadotropic hypogonadism results from inadequate testicular exposure to endogenous gonadothrophins, usually both FSH and LH.

Fertile eunuch syndrome in which there is isolated deficiency of LH. Spermatogenesis seems to proceed normally but virilization is inadequate as a result of insufficient androgen exposure.

In male subfertility where there is isolated deficiency of FSH.

In certain males poor sperm production may be because of abnormalities in biosynthesis of testosterone by Leydig cells.

Sertoli cells play major role in nutrition and deficiency or inadequate stimulation of these cells play major role in deficient spermatogenesis.

In many males there may be idiopathic Oligoa-zoospermia as there is no demonstrable cause to point out.

Deficiency can be corrected by giving appropriate hormone to him in appropriate dose.

ANDROGENS TESTOSTERONE

Testosterone is poorly absorbed after oral intake.

Parenteral form of testosterone Phenyl propionates, long acting testosterone emanate or mixture of both are used for injections.

Esters are injected and physician can see high concentration of testosterone in blood and this remains in blood for 3 to 5 days and during this time there is suppression of LHRH, LH, and FSH.

These cause spermatogenesis at decreased stage and this method is used for suppression of spermatogenesis.

ANDROGEN DERIVATIVES

In literature people have tried so many derivatives and particularly available in markets are Mesterolone stable derivative and can be taken orally.

Mesterolone in dose of 75 mg/day and even high dose of 150 mg/day does not give promising results.

Testosterone undecanoate is non-toxic testosterone derivative and well absorbed after oral administration and effect is seen by increase amount of 5a-dihydrotestosterone in peripheral blood. This molecule has minimal effect on hypothalamo pituitary function.

Dose is 120 mg/day.

This is very good drug for patients with Idiopathic oligospermia and effect can be seen by increase in live sperm.

HUMAN GONADOTHROPHINS

Physicians have now variety of gonadothrophins in their hand like hMG combination of FSH and LH; pure FSH with hCG (chorionic gonadothrophins).

These all are found very useful in case of Hypogonadotropic hypogonadism.

In patients with idiopathic oligospermia pure FSH is found very useful and give very promising result in patients with poor sperm quality.

LHRH (LUTENIZING HORMONE RELEASING HORMONE)

LHRH has been used by portable computerized pump for infusion and gives very good results in patients with Hypogonadotropic hypogonadism of hypothalamic origin.

Nasal or subcutaneous high dose may suppress both hormonogenesis and spermatogenesis.

Treatment by interfering with estradiol.

Physician can interfere with effect of estradiol either by inhibition of its synthesis by means of aromatous inhibitor or through blocking its effect on target cell by means of antiestrogen.

Testolctine, a potent aromatous inhibitor, has given little positive result in small group of study.

Antiestrogens are widely used with promising results. Physicians are using Clomiphene citrate, a racemic mixture of both isomers, which gives a significant intrinsic estrogenic activity in addition to its dominant antiestrogenic effect.

In large study of 3362 cycles with 875 patients, 41% is the pregnancy rate with 25 days cycle in male with dose of 25 mg/day.

Tamoxifen is also used in male in dose of 20 mg/day which have only anti-estrogenic effect. This substance stimulates the hypothalamus and releases LHRH by setting the threshold of feedback at higher levels. As a result the secretion of LH, FSH and testosterone go upto 60 and 100%. Use of drug for 4 to 6 months definitely gives very good outcome.

CHAPTER 7

Surgical Approach for Male Infertility

Today in arena of ART (Artificial reproductive technique), beautiful art of microsurgical technique for male infertility, opens new door for the males and they can become father with only one sperm derived from their seminiferous tubules and can become normospermic by technique of vasoepididyomopalsty.

Microsurgical repair evolves from an almost classic surgical discipline, e.g. microsurgical repair of vasectomy, to a high tech discipline where the surgeon's skill combines traditional surgical technique with the understanding of procedure to obtain spermatozoa for fertilization by microinjection into mature oocyte.

Although reproductive andrology has come almost completely under the ever-widening opportunities of IVF, there remains a distinct place for operating andrologist, both, within and outside the field of IVF.

It is inconceivable that the microsurgeon trying to obtain vital spermatozoa from an obstructed tract, should not be acquainted with the normal anatomy, physiology and pathology of male adnexa.

SURGICAL APPROACH TOWARDS MALE

First, we have to be good clinician and find out the case which patient will require scrotal exploration and will get good benefit out of it (Fig. 7.1).

Mostly scrotal exploration is done in cases of vasectomy reversal, palpable head of epididymis suggesting obstruction and in cases with palpable vas deference.

Mostly in men with azoospermia, normal testes and/or normal FSH, one encounters normal spermatogenesis but presence of epididymal or vasal obstruction.

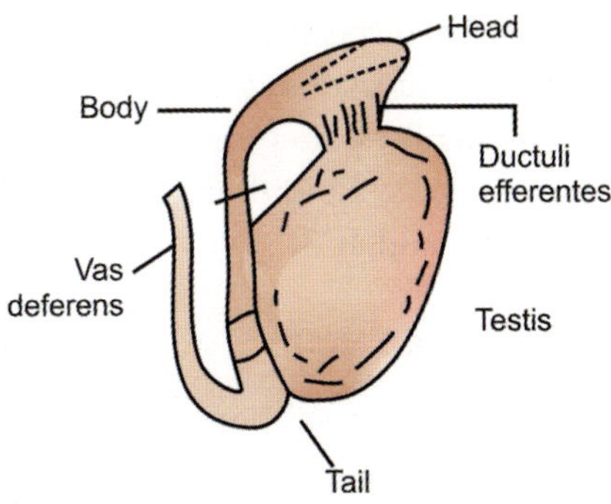

Fig. 7.1: Scrotal exploration

These may be due to congenital or posttraumatic obstruction or Young's syndrome. When microsurgical repair is impossible, one should imply the possibility of epididymal or testicular retrieval.

In doubtful cases in which we find a low ejaculate volume, low pH and undetectable fructose and we want to confirm congenital absence of vas we have to go for scrotal exploration.

We have to be very cautious in taking decision of scrotal exploration particularly in cases of oligoazoospermia due to alleged subobstruction. The cumulative results of IVF and/or techniques of assisted fertilization are probably better than those of reconstructive microsurgery, which may in turn make male into azoospermic.

Other big group of patients with vericocele becomes candidate for scrotal exploration. One remaining indication for scrotal exploration is persistent azoospermia even after vasectomy repair. In this instance one may attempt a second vasovasostomy.

In any case, careful inspection of the degree of dilatation of the epididymal tubular system may be helpful in determining whether the patients can become a candidate for MESA (Microscopic Epididymal Sperm Aspiration) combined with IVF and ICSI.

OPERATIVE SCROTOTOMY

Like any operation this operation should be done with appropriate anesthesia. Usually we prefer to do it in general anesthesia with all instruments ready for reconstructive microsurgery. This include operative microscope, skillful assistant and light microscope to examine slides for presence of motile spermatozoa and in some rare cases we have to go for preoperative radiography also.

Scrotum is opened by standard incision horizontal or vertical.

All findings are recorded on a preprinted drawing of the scrotum which can be helpful in explaining to the patients and the referring physician also.

This documentation is very useful in case of MESA to know the area of tubular dilatation.

After completion of procedure both tunica vaginalis and skin are stitched separately and patient can be discharged on next day asking for follow-up for stitch removal.

Now in era of endoscopy we are also performing scrotal endoscopy and has got very good advantage of vedio image over printed report for better understandings.

PATHOLOGY AT SCROTUM

Testis is palpated first and slight is weak consistency or decreased size may suggest absent or decreased spermatogenesis.

All biopsy specimens of testis should be taken into Bouin or Stieve solution.

Parameters of histological evaluation of testicular biopsy:

1. Number of seminiferous tubules containing germinal cells (mature spermatids, early round spermatids, arrest at spermatocyte stage, arrest at spermatogenic stage).
2. Number of tubules without germinal cells (Sertoli cell only, no seminiferous epithelium).
3. Tubular diameters (minimum, maximum, mean).
4. Thickness of germinal tissue (Mean of radial basement).
5. Distribution, localization and morphology of spermatogonia.
6. Spermatocyte morphology and distribution.
7. Spermatids morphology and distribution.
8. Degenerating cells
9. Sertoli cell description.
10. Leydig cell description.
11. Special findings, e.g. tumor cells.

Epididymis is carefully examined using magnifying optics for identification of obstructive sites. If testicular biopsy reveals spermatogenesis then microsurgical repair is usually indicated surgical option.

If dilatation appears to be less pronounced and at different levels of the tubular system, the chance of having a very diseased tubular system is very high and surgical outcome of vasoepididymostomy is very poor.

Usually we encounter single or congenital epididymal cysts, hematic cyst, congenital anomalies of the testiculo epididymal junction, spermatocele, epididymal dystrophy, and empty epididymis syndrome.

Fluid in tunica vaginalis acts as replica of what happens in the interstitial or even intratubular compartment of the testis, same as, fluid in POD (Pouch of Douglas) reflects activity of cyclical ovarian function.

Studies of fluid of tunica vaginalis show very high androgen concentration.

High concentration of antibodies of Chlamydia is seen in patients with idiopathic oligoazoospermia.

REANASTOMOSIS OF VAS DEFERENS

In last few years this technique has increased because of there is increased rate of vasectomy and after few years man can change their minds.

Reasons for reanastomosis like:

1. Frequency of divorce
2. Second marriage
3. Because of sound financial condition they can afford one more child
4. Loss of one child.

Couple usually asks whether there is any chance of defective baby, after reversal.

We have to counsel the patients that this operation is techniqually difficult and must tell them regarding percentage of success of procedure and pain he has to bare same as that of vasectomy.

We have to clarify following critical points:
1. The anastomosis must be made at level where sperms are present.
2. The anastomosis must remain patent.
3. Fertility depends on securing not merely a good number of sperms but an adequate number of motile sperms.
4. Most of the time fertility is not immediate and a time interval is necessary, before sperms are present in adequate numbers for impregnation.

CHOICE OF OPERATION

Depending on the finding of sperms at the time of surgery, one of two surgical procedures is performed or a combination of one procedure on one side and another on the other side.

If sperm, or sperm head, are seen, in the spermatic fluid, emerging when the testicular end of the vas is opened, a vasovasostomy is performed.

If no fluid can be expressed, or if the fluid fails to show sperm on repeated examination, the tunica vaginalis should be opened and epididymis inspected.

Dilated tubules at the caput of the epididymis, with empty tubules below, indicate obstruction at that junction. An epididymotomy is performed and emerging fluid contains sperms, an epididymovasostomy is performed to allow the testis to contribute these sperm to the semen.

Operating surgeon must be capable of doing either of operation and we must inform patients and must take written consent for whichever procedure we can do on him which gives better result to him.

Choice of operation room with all emergencies is ideal but literature shows that some surgeon take it as OPD procedure and doing in local anesthesia with some sedation in well-equipped office but decision should be individualized.

PREPARATION OF THE PATIENTS

As before any operation pre-operative assessment is necessary like all investigations and history of bleeding tendency, medication for some diseases like DM, HT or any others.

As majority of reversal cases are of young patients so in local anesthesia it would not be a big problem during surgery.

Preoperative examination is of utmost importance and we must ask for the interval between vasectomy and reversal time as incidence of epididymal obstruction is increased with time.

REPAIR OF STERILIZATION (VASOVASOSTOMY)

Vasovasostomy for repair of sterilization is now the most frequent and rewarding contribution for operating andrologist to make in post-testicular obstruction.

As there is increase frequency of vasectomy and divorce, the requirement of reversal of sterilization is increasing with time.

As female reversal is *little more difficult than male reversal, technique of ART is taken up by.*

Failures of reversal are candidate for donor insemination or by some technique of ART through testis like retrieval of spermatozoa from epidydimis.

Vasovasostomy is low impact operation and remain as first choice than directly going for ART.

We must counsel patients regarding success of reversal as high titer of antibodies will reduce chance of pregnancy.

Complete gynecological examination of female is must as soon as semen becomes positive for sperms as these group of females are usually not very young and may be suffering form subfertility or irregular periods or anovulation.

If antibodies are high in titer and on examination poor sperm characteristics are present and couple is not able to conceive after one year of reversal we have to go for ART.

TECHNIQUE OF VASOVASOSTOMY

The incision for vasovasostomy should be of adequate length to allow good exposure of both end of vas.

Prostatic stump may be embedded in fibrous tissue in the lower inguinal region. It may be necessary to extend incision upto inguinal ligament, sometimes it is very difficult to identify the vasectomy site and sometimes it is very easy.

Sperm granuloma is usually found at testicular end and this is very bad prognostic factor affecting patency.

By dissection of adjacent tissues both ends of vas are freed and constant irrigation should be done by warm saline by micro IV set.

Prostatic end is flushed with saline to assess patency. For epididymal end just take fluid or if it does not come by itself just massage testicular end and look under microscopic examination for presence of spermatids or motile spermatozoa. Even sometimes, no fluid is coming from testicular ends then one should perform a vasoepididymostomy linking the vas to the transition zone between the caput and the corpus.

If there appears to be no obstruction at all, there is probably an underlying testicular factor.

We must be very good documentor and excellent drawing person because records are very good friends.

We must be very careful regarding nerves, blood vessels (vascular) and lymphatics.

Technique of perfect anastomosis is not enough to restore the contractile function of vas deferens. To make lower epididymis functional, vascularization is utmost important as vascularization is not perfect testicular necrosis may sometimes occur.

We must follow the guidelines described in microsurgical technique for suturing stumps of vessel ends. Proline 4/0 is used for suturing and both stumps should "kiss" either by side-to-side or end-to-end anastomosis.

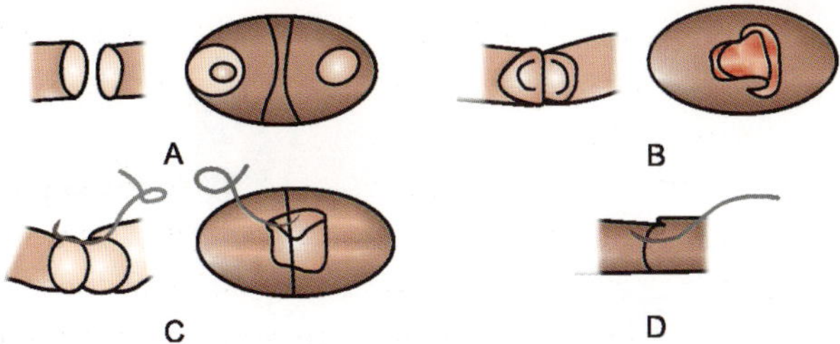

Fig. 7.2A to D: Two-layer technique

There are two popular methods for suturing—single layer or two layers. Single layer is fast and fantastic in experienced hands to feel symmetry at both the ends (Figs 7.2A to D).

Two layer technique is best for the ends having disparity in diameter.

Usually 6/0 Prolene is used for one layer anastomosis and 8/0 are preferably for the mucosal anastomosis.

Lets talk regarding new technique of applying fibrin glue as an adjuvant but still it is in experimental stages. Some surgeons are using stents but this is not generally accepted.

Scrotum is then closed in layers, postoperative antibiotics, and antiinflammatory drugs for 7 days and bed rest for 48 hours.

Usually all these patients are encouraged to ejaculate as early as possible.

A first sperm sample should be requested at 10-14 days, azoospermia does not exclude patency later on, and presence of spermatozoa proves patency and fantastic outcome.

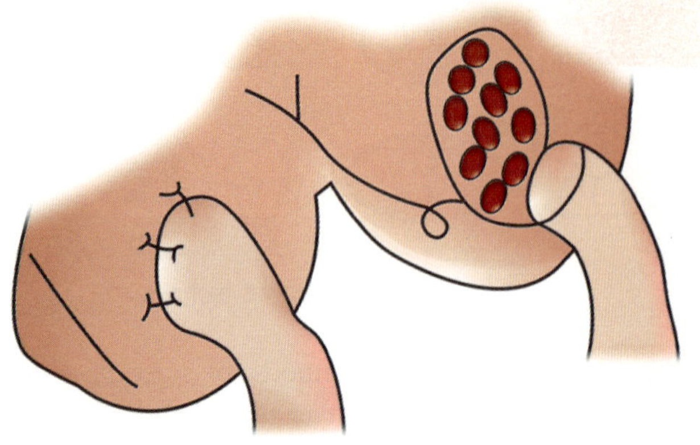

Fig. 7.3: High vasoepididymostomy

REPAIR OF EPIDIDYMAL BLOCK

Nowadays this technique is not much in use, due to decrease in incidence of gonorrheic epidydimitis, which usually causes a well-localized low block and clear dilatation of the caput (Fig. 7.3).

In high vasoepididymostomy, the vas is connected to the level of rete testis of the efferent ducts.

Chapter 8

Newer Drug

CO-ENZYME Q10

Infertility affects more than 80 million people worldwide.

In India, according to WHO report, primary and secondary infertility account for 3% and 8%.

Studies of infertile couple in India reveal that infertility is life crisis and stressful experience with invisible losses.

Male infertility is one of the most common, identifiable causes of human reproduction failure.

Male related disorders are present in upto 50% of child less couples and would be perceived as a particular threat to conventional views of masculinity.

More than 90% of male infertility accounts for poor sperm quality and motility (Tables 8.1 and 8.2).

Table 8.1: Normal semen analysis

Parameters	*Values*
Ejaculate volume	1.5-5.0 ml
Sperm density	> 20 million/ml
Sperm motility	> 60%
Forward progression	> 2 (Scale of 1-4)
Morphology	> 30% (WHO criteria) > 14% (Strict criteria)

Table 8.2: Subcategory of male infertility factor

Subcategory	*Motility (%)*	*Morphology (% Normal)*
Mild	40-50	30-40
Moderate	20-40	10-30
Severe	< 20	<10

Table 8.3: Terminology

Azoospermia = no sperm in semen
Oligopsermia = very few sperm in semen, < 20 x 10^6/ml
Severe oligopsermia = < 5 x 10^6/ml
Asthenospermia = poor motility of sperm
Teratospermia = abnormal sperm forms < 30% (WHO) < 14% (Kruger)

DECLINING SPERM COUNT

Since last 50 years numerous studies shows constant decline in mean sperm density and seminal volume (Table 8.3).

Carlsen et al analyzed 61 studies including 14,947 men for mean sperm density and mean volume. Results showed significant decline in mean sperm density from 113 million/ml to 66 million/ml and volume average of 3.40 to 2.75 ml.

Main culprits for 20% drop in volume and 58% decline in sperm production are over exposure to environmental toxins, chemicals and infection. They can reduce sperm count either by direct effects on testicular function or on the hormone systems.

The primary suspects in the link between environmental assaults and infertility are reactive oxygen species (ROS) also called oxidants.

OXIDATIVE STRESS AND SPERM ABNORMALITIES

Defective sperm function in infertile men has been associated with:

- ROS induced sperm damage (by increased lipid peroxidation) and

- Impaired function of antioxidant defences in spermatozoa.

ROS plays an important role in sperm physiological functions and elevated levels of ROS or oxidative stresses are know to impair sperm cell function and play a negative role in male factor fertility.

Pasqualotto FF, Shrama RK, et al conducted a study in 169 infertile patients to determine whether particular semen characteristics in various clinical diagnoses of infertility are associated with high oxidative stress and whether any group of infertile men is more likely to have seminal oxidative stress. They concluded that irrespective of the clinical diagnosis and semen characteristics, the presence of seminal oxidative stress in infertile men suggest its role in the pathophysiology of infertility.

CO-ENZYME Q10 (UBIQUINONE) IN MALE INFERTILITY

A multi faceted therapeutic approach to improve male fertility involves:

- Correcting oxidative stress to encourage optimal sperm production and
- Improving sperm motility and function.

Co-enzyme Q10, fat soluble quinine first identified in 1957, has proven beneficial in treating male infertility in the above aspects.

Co-enzyme Q10 is an energy promoting agent and antioxidant associated with membrane and lipoproteins. The reduce form of co-enzyme Q10 biosynthesis is markedly active in testis and high levels of its reduced form (QH2) are present in semen that suggest its protective role as a scavenger in this biological system.

Co-enzyme Q10 prevents lipid peroxidation in the sperm membranes.

Furthermore since sperm production and function are highly energy-dependent processes, deficiency of co-enzyme Q10, a component of the mitochondrial respiratory chain that plays a crucial role in energy metabolism and adenosine triphosphate (ATP) generation could presumably be a contributing factor to infertility in men.

In sperm cell, the majority of co-enzyme is concentrated in the mitochondria of the mid piece where it is involved in energy production. Thus the energy-dependent process in the sperm cell depends on the availability of co-enzyme Q10.

RATIONALE FOR TREATMENT

Present data suggest that sperm cells, characterized by low motility and abnormal morphology, have low levels of co-enzyme Q10 while high intracellular concentrations of co-enzyme Q10 may represent a mechanism of protection of spermatozoa.

Balercia G, Arnaldi G, et al determined levels of co-enzyme Q10 and of its reduced and oxidized forms (QH2, Ubiquinol/Qox, ubiquinone) in sperm and seminal plasma of asthenozoospermic patients and of controls. The results have shown significant lower levels of co-enzyme Q10 and of its reduced forms, QH2, in semen samples from patients with asthenospermia: furthermore the co-enzyme Q10 content was mainly associated with spermatozoa. The present data suggest that the QH2/Qox ratio may be an index of oxidative stress and its reduction is a risk factor for semen quality. Sperm cells with low levels of co-enzyme are less capable in dealing with oxidative stress which could lead to a reduced QH2/Qox ratio.

Alleva R, Scararmucci, et al assessed co-enzyme Q10 content in both the reduced and oxidized from (Ubiquinol/ Ubiquinone) and hydroperoxidase levels in seminal plasma and seminal fluid form 32 subjects with a history of infertility.

Results showed

- Significant co-relation between ubiquinol content and sperm count in seminal plasma.
- An inverse co-relation between ubiquinol content and hydroperoxidase levels both in seminal plasma and in seminal fluids.
- A strong co-relation among sperm count, motility and ubiquinol-10 content seminal fluid.
- An inverse co-relation between ubiquinol/ubiquinone ratio and percentage of abnormal morphology.

These results suggest that ubiquinol-10 inhibits hydroperoxidase formation in seminal fluid and in seminal plasma. Since peroxidation in sperm cells is an important factor affecting male infertility, Ubiquinol could assume a diagnostic and/or a therapeutic role in these patients.

Mancicni A De Marinis Assayed co-enzyme Q10 levels in total seminal fluid or both, in seminal fluids and seminal plasma, in 77 subjects with normal or pathological findings at standard semen analysis. Co-enzyme Q10 levels showed a significant co-relation with sperm counts and with sperm motility. This data suggests a pathological meaning of co-enzyme Q10 in human seminal fluids. Co-enzyme Q10 measurements could represent an important examination in infertile patients; moreover from these results a rationale arose for treatment with exogenous co-enzyme.

Tanimura J showed a study which showed that administration of co-enzyme Q10 resulted in a considerable increase sperm count and motility in group of infertile men.

So, physician can consider it as rational treatment of oligopsermia.

Lewin A, Lavon H performed a study to evaluate the effect of co-enzyme Q10 on sperm motility *in vitro*, after incubation of 38 samples of asthenospermic and normal motility sperm and *in vivo* in 17 patients with low fertilization rates. Increase in motility was observed in the sperm from asthenospermic men and a significant improvement was noted in fertilization rates. It was concluded that the administration of co-enzyme Q10 may result in improvement in sperm functions.

Exogenous administration of co-enzyme Q10 may play a positive role in the treatment of infertile men with idiopathic asthenospermia, according to results of study published in the 2004 January issue of fertility and sterility.

Study of Balercia G, Mosca F clarifies a potential role of co-enzyme Q10 in infertile men with asthenoazoospermia. Co-enzyme Q10 was administered orally. Semen sample were collected at baseline and after 6 months of therapy. Results showed that:

- Co-enzyme Q10 levels increase significantly in seminal plasma and in sperm after treatment

- A significant increase was also found in sperm cell motility as confirmed by CASA (Computer assisted analysis).

It was concluded that the exogenous administration of co-enzyme Q10 might play a positive role in the treatment of asthenoazoospermia.

This is probably the result of its role in mitochondrial bioenergetics and its antioxidant properties.

DOSAGE

Self-emulsifying drug delivery systems can be used for the design of formulation in order to improve the oral absorption of lipophylic drug compounds like co-enzyme Q10. Soft gelatin capsules provide good emulsion and absorption.

Usual dose of Co-enzyme Q10 is 60-120 mg per day.

SAFETY

Co-enzyme Q10 is generally well tolerated and no serious adverse effects have been reported with long-term use.

Overvad K, Diamant B reviewed literature concerning Co-enzyme Q10. No important adverse effects were reported from experiments using daily supplements of Q10, upto 200 mg for 6-12 months and 100 mg daily for upto 6 years.

In series of 5143 patients treated with 30 mg/day of co-enzyme Q10, the following of side effects were reported:

- Epigastric discomfort 0.39%
- Loss of appetite 0.23%
- Nausea 0.16%
- Diarrhea 0.12%

Co-enzyme Q10 supplementation is an effective and safe addition in the armamentarium of therapies available in the battle against male infertility, a disorder with not only medical but psychosocial implication.

Chapter 9

Artificial Insemination and IUI

Insemination means deposition of semen in vagino-cervical region. If it occurs in natural way it is called natural insemination. Instrumental deposition of semen in genital canal is called artificial insemination. This term can be extended depending on the source of semen.

When the sperms used are of husband it is Artificial Insemination of Husband's sperms (AIH).

If the source of sperms is other than husband's it is Artificial Insemination of Donor's sperms (AID).

In 1790 John Hunter suggested a patient of hypospadias to deposit his own semen into his wife's vagina. Repeated attempts resulted in pregnancy. This is the first documented case.

The first reported human donor insemination (AID) was performed in 1884 by William Pancoast. The indication was azoospermia of her husband. The semen was collected from a hired man and was injected in vagina under anesthesia.

Faulty semino-cervical contact due to anatomical abnormalities in either partner may be corrected by artificial placing of the semen. A hostile uterincervix can be treated by intrauterine insemination.

NATURAL NORMAL MECHANISM

Sperms deposited in vas are not motile until they meet fluid from seminal vesicle.

Sexual intercourse, done during the proper days ends up with proper ejaculation. Semen deposited in posterior fornix mixes with vaginal secretion having acidic pH ranging from 4.2 to 4.7 and then. Propagation of sperms-

chemotaxis, to cervical canal—which has alkaline pH of 7.0 to 7.5.

Quality of cervical mucus is very important. In pre ovulatory days' mucus is thin, watery, and clear with high elasticity. This is favorable cervical mucus. Through cervical canal sperms will migrate towards endometrial cavity, where they are capacitated and through corneal end of fallopian tube enter the ampular region of tube.

Similar simultaneous event takes place in female genital tract. Dominent follicle ruptures at LH surge and ovulation occurs. Fimbria of the fallopian tube covers the whole ovary in umbrella fashion and sucks the oocyte and make it travel to ampulla.

Oocyte is then surrounded by sperms. One of the sperms enters through corona radiata and makes the oocyte fertilized. This fertilized ovum travels to endometrial cavity and nidation take place for further pregnancy.

So for natural events to occurs the requirements are:

1. Proper ejaculation of semen
2. Enough quantity and quality of sperms
3. Proper atmosphere at cervical opening (favorable cervical mucus)
4. Normal patent tube
5. Prepared endometrium
6. Timed ovulation
7. Proper ovum pick-up.
8. Sperm penetration to oocyte
9. Proper nidation of fertilized ovum.

Anything wrong occoured at anyone of the stages, pregnancy does not occur.

If anything is wrong in above first four criteria it may lead to the need of instrumental deposition of sperms in cervical canal or endometrial cavity meaning AIH /AID/ IUI.

INDICATIONS

1. Ejaculatory disorders

   No proper sexual intercourse and/or absence of ejaculations.

   Absence of ejaculations may be psychogenic or organic like spinal cord injuries.

   Medical disorders like DM or Multiple Sclerosis.

   Anatomic reasons like hypospadias or Neuorogenic like retrograde ejaculations.

2. Hostile cervical mucus

   Thick-viscous

   less elastic

3. Male factors

   Improper seminal fluid or semen report like

   Aspermia, Azoospermia,

   Oligospermia, Asthenozoospermia.

   less motility or absent

   Necrosospermia-dead spermatozoa

   Oligoazoospermia-less spermatozoa.

4. Acidic or presence of ASA

   Antisperm antibody in Male or Female serum or semen or cervical mucus.

5. Unexplained
6. Combination of more then one.

SELECTION OF PATIENT

Criteria: Ejaculatory failures, Poor post coital results, Sperm problems, unexplained infertility.

Requirements: Age of female, preferable less than 40 years and otherwise normal.

COUNSELING

It is the key part for taking up the procedure and for successful result.

Proper explanation of the need to do it and its success rates, procedures included should be discussed in details with the couple. If couple has to be co-operative, Doctor has to be considerable. All quarries of couple should be clarified including cost involved.

Cycle Regulation

The idea is to get mature oocyte at expected time.

A course of Antibiotics and down regulation in previous cycle.

Proper induction of ovulation by CC, HMG, FSH, hCG

Proper monitoring of ovulation by TVS and Serum estradiol levels.

SEMEN PREPARATION

Ideally it is an expertise job and left it to SPERM BANK.

Antibiotics to male partner in previous cycle to clear any seminal fluid infection.

Collection-minimum 3 days abstinence.

By Masturbation.

Collect in wide, clean, sterile glass dish. Transfer to sperm bank in one hour.

If donor's semen is to use then—Donor should be unknown to couple, physically and mentally resemble to husband-Blood group matching-No STD-and fertile count and motility.

AIH (ARTIFICIAL INSEMINATION HUSBAND)

Consent

It is mandatory to take prior consent and information regarding AIH.

Patients (couple) must be informed regarding infrequent success, limitation of procedure.

There are all chances of failure of semen sample on demand.

Success rate totally depends on selection of patient with regular ovulatory cycle, and adequate luteal phase patency of tube.

Cycle is monitored with USG and on day of ovulation insemination should be carried out.

Sample

Husband should supply semen as either whole or split ejaculate.

Different routes for insemination are intracervical, intrauterine and intravaginal, depending on quality of sample received.

Posterior fornix, depends on quality of sample received.

In cases of washed sample by swim-up or per coil gradient it always should be done by IUI only.

Whole semen sample should be deposited in posterior fornix, or intracervical by cervical cap.

Timing for AIH

Very much important issue because it is very difficult for the husband that he is not capable of doing the act and psychological disturbance is on its top.

We are monitoring cycle by USG and patient is already on ovulation inducing drugs (Figs 9.1 and 9.2).

AIH should be planned on the day of ovulation either spontaneous or induced by hCG injection and done twice at interval of 24 hours.

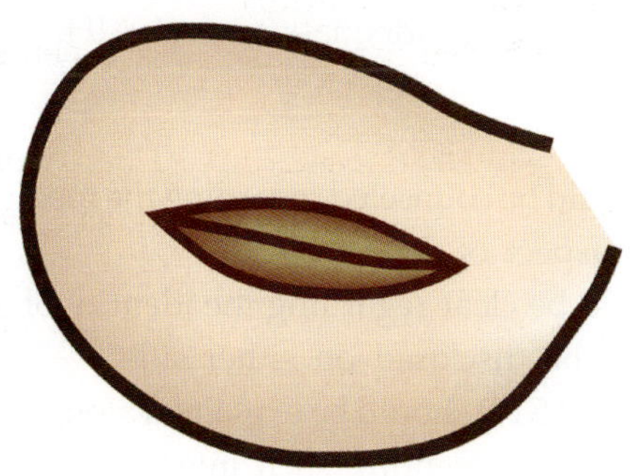

Fig. 9.1: USG-secretory phase

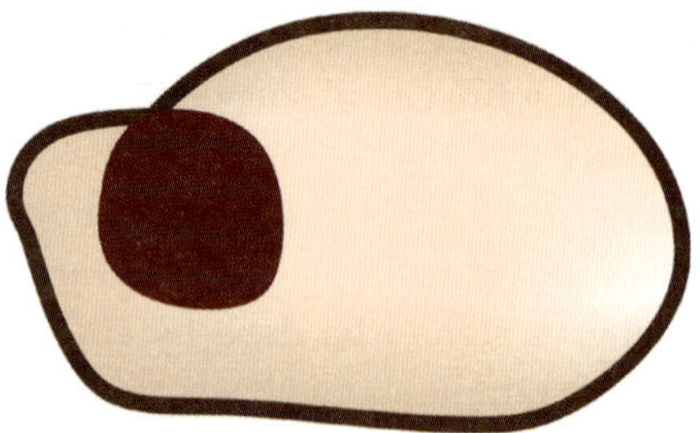

Fig. 9.2: USG-mature follicle

Result

Usually patient will conceive in first four to six cycles of insemination.

Failure may be because of underlying pathology like endometriosis, peritubal periovarian diseases, LPD.

AID (ARTIFICIAL INSEMINATION DONOR)

Donor insemination should be offered to couple with azoospermia and oligoasthenoteratospermia who fail to conceive despite an adequate trial of AIH.

Consent

Couple should be counseled regarding the medical, ethical, and legal aspect of AID.

It should be clear regarding the identity of donor and should not be disclosed on either side.

The risk of STD should be explained along with utmost care taken for preventing such infection.

Risk of developing birth defect will remain same as with couple conceiving spontaneously.

Donor recipient anonymity should be discussed.

DONOR SCREENING

Donor is interviewed for reliability, availability and psychological stability.

First step is history taking with all details of medical and genetic disorders of donor and first blood relatives.

Artificial insemination of donor can be:

- Intravaginal
- Intracervical
- Intrauterine

First two procedures are simple and almost all doctors do it routinely.

IUI needs proper set up and understanding

For IV or IC- Intravaginal-Intracervical—Clean vagina with saline- Semen is taken in small but long syringe-Best done in lithotomy position of patient.

Proper deposition of seminal fluid is done at cervical canal-opening and in posterior fornix. Cervical cap can be used after it to prevent regurgitation.

IUI (INTRAUTERINE INSEMINATION)

The term IUI defines the deposition of sperms in the uterine cavity by means of catheter or special IUI cannula that has been passed through the cervical canal. In this way, an increased number of sperm cells can be brought instantaneously to the proximity of fertilized site. And cervical barrier can be by-passed. The reduction in the content of seminal plasma, that contains inhibitors of fertilization and prostaglandins, is associated advantage of the IUI procedure (Figs 9.3A and B).

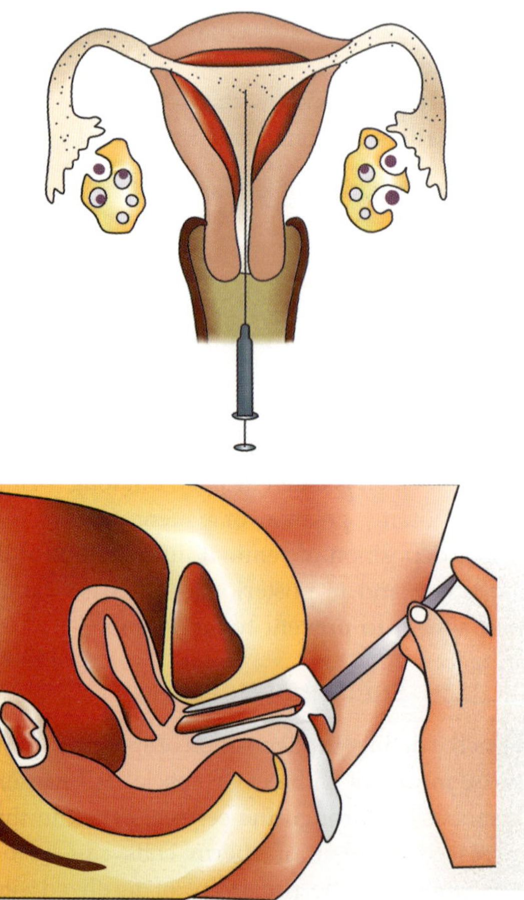

Figs 9.3A and B: IUI procedures

Usually semen sample prepared in laboratory and send to clinician (Figs. 9.4A and B).

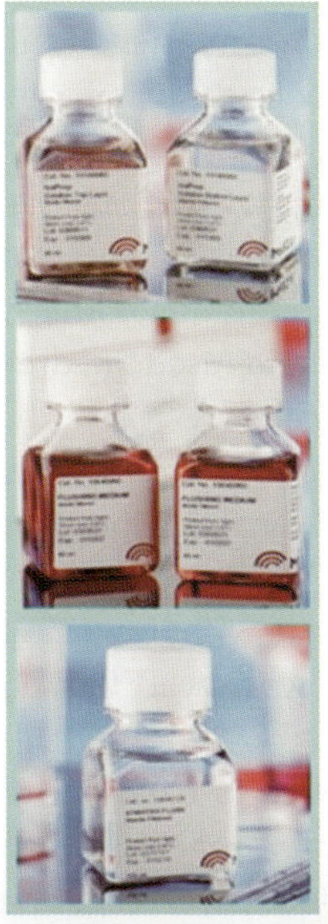

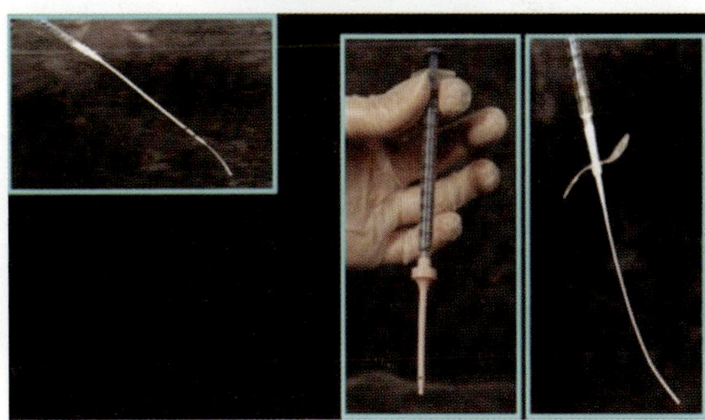

Figs 9.4A and B: A. Different media. B. Different connula for IUI

The volume of insemination is around 1 to 4 ml according to technique used for preparation of sample.

The woman lies in the lithotomy position on table.

A warm speculum is moistened with warm sterile water and gently inserted in the vagina to expose cervix and cervical os.

The cervix is gently washed or wiped with several cotton balls shocked in normal saline solution.

The insemination cannula is attached to the tuberculin or insulin syringe and used in drawing-up the sperm suspension (Fig. 9.5).

The cannula is gently introduced into the uterine cavity through the cervical canal and the sperm suspension gently expelled.

All instruments are withdrawn and the patient allowed to lay on the table with head low position before going home.

We usually advice to have one intercourse after IUI at night. No literature support is available for that practice but it gives tremendous psychological support to the patient that they might have conceived with act they had done around ovulation.

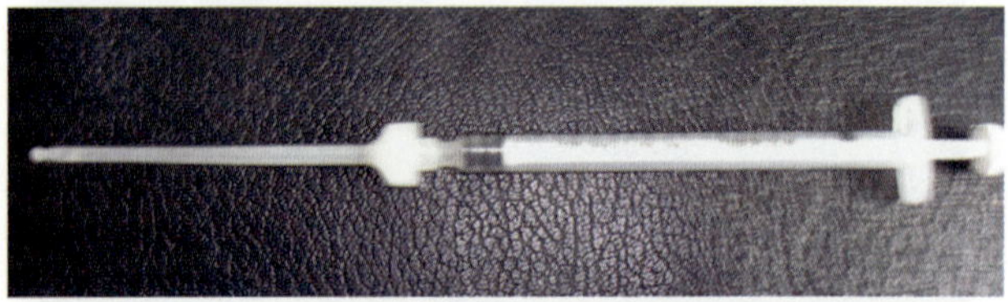

Fig. 9.5: IUI cannula with tuberculin syringe

Success Rate

About 10-15% of couple will become pregnant in each cycle of treatment.

Higher rates about 34% have been reported by some centre.

Mostly three or four IUI cycles will give very good results.

Complications

Not so common in IUI cycle.

Pelvic infection may occur in 0.01 to 0.2%.

Allergic reaction to albumin, antibiotics or some other components of the sperm culture medium.

Multiple pregnancies increased upto 11-30%.

It is not yet clear if IUI leads to the formation of antisperm antibodies in the female.

Incidence of abortion is between 20-30%. Ectopic pregnancy is around 3-4%.

CHAPTER 10

Assisted Reproductive Technology (ART)

With advance technology of ART now it is boon for males who are not able to conceive by natural ways.

If you see in the normal individual, millions of sperms are deposited in posterior vagina but plenty of them are not able to gain access into cervix.

Out of lucky ones who enter into the cervix and then uterine cavity, only few thousands are strong enough to enter into the lumen of tube.

Ovum is waiting in the garden of ampulla and the strongest of them get attached around the zona and fuse with the oolema after passing perivitteline space and undergo the acrosomal reaction.

At the same time, a chemical reaction takes place in the oocyte with formation of cortical granules to prevent polyspermia.

To achieve this success the sperm should be morphologically normal and must have sufficient energy to penetrate zona pellucida.

So *in vivo* chance of fertility is very low or drastically down in cases of lows motility, low count and so on.

IUI becomes boon to those couples with problems of low count and motility as we have discussed different methods of preparation of sperm media for different individuals so we can offer this to those large class of patients who can be benefited without going into more expensive ART.

In ART, also minimum requirement of spermatozoa will be 50000-100000. So we have to prepare sperm for this technique also.

DEVELOPMENT OF MICROSURGICAL FERTILIZATION

In vitro the zona pellucida is the major barrier for penetration into the eggs by spermatozoa.

Using micromanipulation technique, this problem can be by passed and it is used since 1914, first by Lillie by injecting sperm into starfish oocyte.

Mitha, et al first reported the clinical application of this technique in 1985 by and 1987 applying the injection of a single spermatozoon in perivitteline space with subsequent fertilization.

TECHNIQUE

Different techniques are available to overcome male sub fertility:

PZD = Partial zona dissection

SUZI = Subzonal insemination

ICSI = Intracytopalsmic sperm injection

All these techniques will require skillful embryologist to perform the task and instrumentation like different micropipette for holding ovum, different microinjection for injecting sperm into the ovum.

We have to make media rich enough to make sperm immotile and we have to catch the sperm looking morphologically normal.

As in ICSI technique, we have to cut the tail of sperm and suck it into the microinjection and then we have to inject it into ovum at 3 o'clock position with aspiration of some fluid from cytoplasm and then again inject into the ovum.

ZONA DRILLING AND PARTIAL ZONA DISSECTION

The idea of drilling holes in the zona pellucida to facilitate access for the spermatozoa to fuse with oolema has been proven successful in different experimental studies (Fig. 10.1).

The zona pellucida may be the most difficult barrier for the penetration process of sperm.

First try to enter into zona was done by digestion of it by acid tyrade solution with micro needle.

This technique had not been so successful in human because of polyspermia.

In 1988, Cohen reported first pregnancy by partial zona dissection by introduction of micropipette tangentially through the zona.

PZD is fairly simple but may impair further development of the embryo because of the potential invasion of

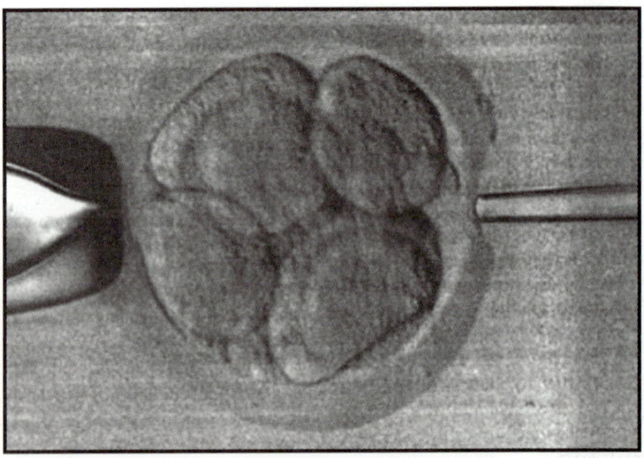

Fig. 10.1: Zona drilling by acid tyrade solution

microorganisms through the gap created, of or cytokines present in the insemination suspension.

SUBZONAL INSEMINATION

In this technique, the zona is not opened but bypassed. After aspiration of a number of spermatozoa into very fine micropipette with an inner diameter of 10 micrometer and beveled at 45 degree, the pipette is passed through the zona with first polar body either at 6 o'clock or 12 o'clock and minimum number of spermatozoa are injected.

After subzonal insemination, only that spermatozoa that which have undergone capacitation and acrosomal reaction are able to fuse with oolema.

Different agents are present for inducing acrosomal reaction such as use of strontium chloride instead of calcium.

However, we had pregnancies without using acrosomal reaction inducing agent and just introducing sperms into perivitteline space.

The occurrence of pregnancy after subzonal insertion of immotile sperm from man with Kartagener syndrome indicates that motility is less obligatory with SUZI than with PZD.

One of the major concerns regarding injection of arbitrarily chosen spermatozoa into perivitteline space may give possibility of increasing incidence of chromosomal abnormality but one study conducted in Monash University shows no increase in chromosomal abnormalities after SUZI fertilized oocyte.

ICSI (INTRACYTOPLASMIC SPERM INJECTION)

The most advanced, most popular and given very good result in terms of carry home baby rate as it will require only one sperm to fertilize the ovum.

In this method, also, natural selection of sperm is lost and we have to select morphologically normal looking sperm into the pipette and inject into the oolema.

The first attempt was made by Lanzendorf in 1988 and it is still very successful method in ART particularly for male sub fertility.

As advancement in this technique is tremendous nowadays, and there is formation of readymade pipette by company and easy to do operation by micromanipulator instrument (Fig. 10.2).

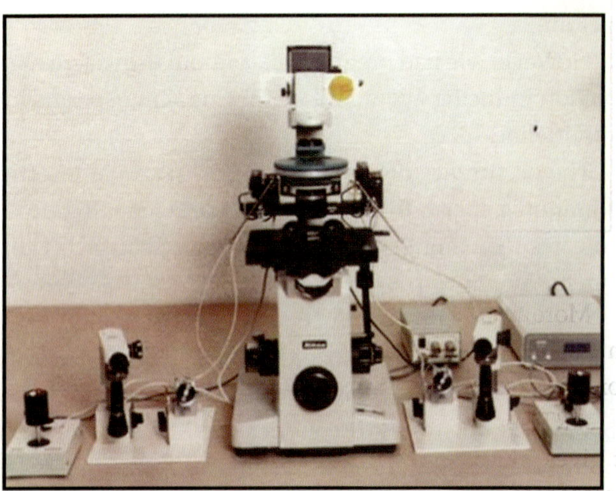

Fig. 10.2: Micromanipulator instruments

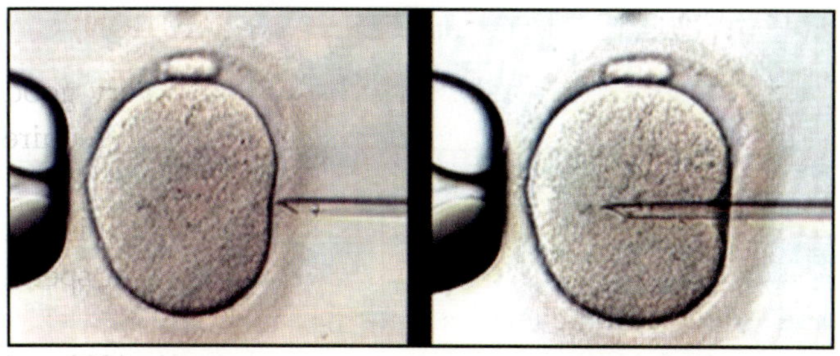

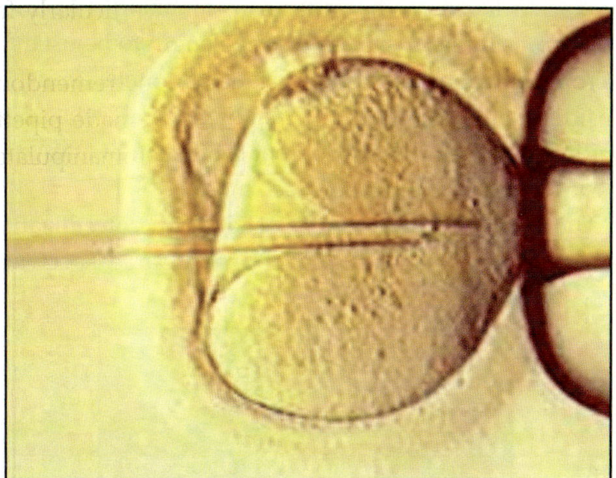

Figs 10.3 and 10.4: ICSI Procedure

More and more embryologist of our country get expertise in this technique and going abroad to do ICSI is proud for us (Figs 10.3 and 10.4).

ART specialists nowadays put more stress on ICSI as it gives more no of 2pn pregnancy and do not rely on acrosomal reaction and can wait for the next day to look for fertilization (Figs 10.6 to 10.9).

Only disadvantage of ICSI at present is cost of micromanipulator and disposable used in process.

FUTURE OF MICROFERTILIZATION TECHNIQUE

Advancement in branch of ART is tremendous. Everyday somebody is doing invention in field to make our job easy and more productive.

Use of LASER in ART is not new but initial use of Nd Yag to Excimer, the progress is amazing (Fig. 10.5).

In choosing laser system or wavelength to be used for microfertilization technique, various parameters must be considered: the danger of thermal damage, the absorbent coefficient of water, the absorbent coefficient of DNA and possibility of use in noncontact mode.

The wavelength that can be used for microfertilization are situated between ultraviolet and infrared spectrum.

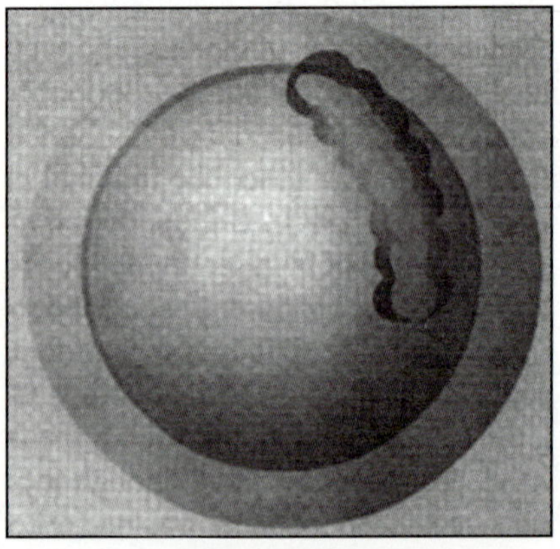

Fig. 10.5: Zona drilling by laser

The possible formation of ablation by-product, in culture medium can exert a toxic effect on development of embryo, can be eliminated by transferring embryo after laser procedure into fresh media.

The absorption spectrum of DNA is at its highest at 200 nm and it is lowest at around 300 nm.

Damage to DNA structure must be prevented and when choosing a laser wavelength for micromanipulation the absorbent spectrum of DNA must be taken into account, although at 308 nm the absorption of DNA is very low.

Another possible use of laser is the removal of extra male pronucleus in the nontouch mode. With the Excimer laser the beam can be focused on the desired target within the zona or cytoplasm and may be used in selective destruction of extra male pronucleus without opening of the zona pellucida and the oolema.

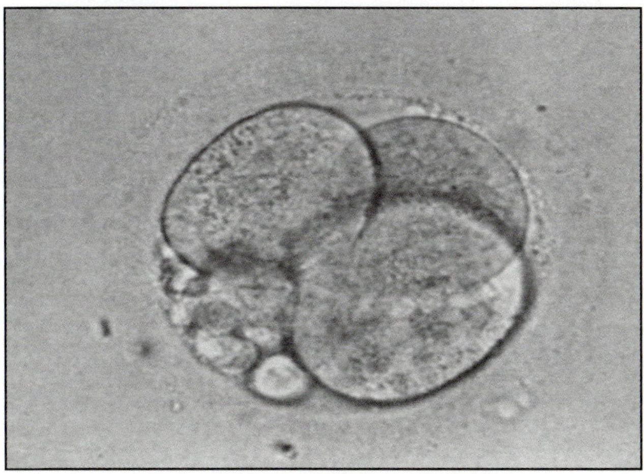

Fig. 10.6: Three-cell embryo

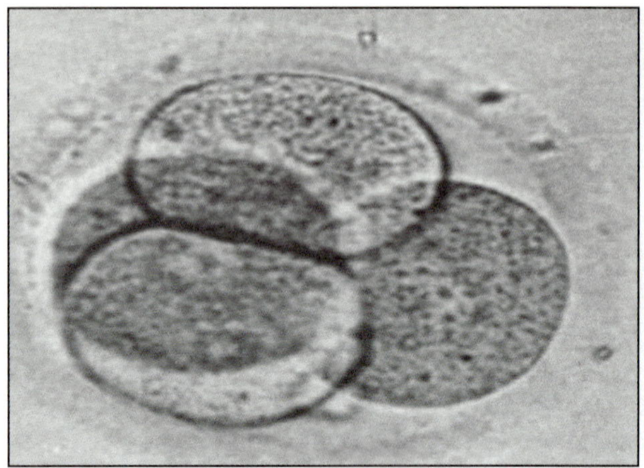

Fig. 10.7: Four-cell embryo

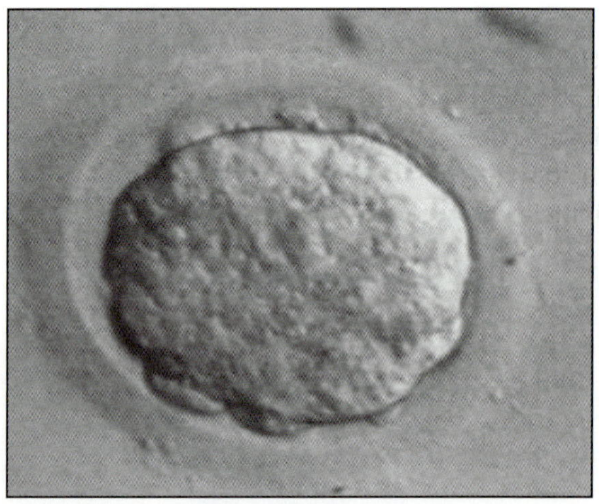

Fig. 10.8: Morula

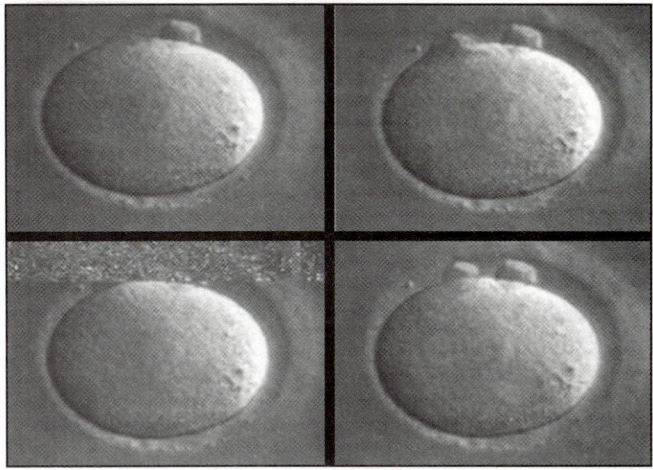

Fig. 10.9: Fertilization

Using the combine UV microbeam (337 nm) and the optical trapping system (Nd Yag 1064 nm) mounted on an inverted microscope, it is possible to open the zona pellucida trapping one spermatozoon and moving into the perivitteline space same time.

Index